Introduction to Public Health

Raymond L. Goldsteen, DrPH, is the Founding Director of the Graduate Program in Public Health and Professor of Preventive Medicine in the School of Medicine at SUNY, Stony Brook. He received his doctoral degree from the Columbia University School of Public Health. He has an extensive background in health care and was formerly a director of health policy research centers at the University of Illinois in Urbana-Champaign, University of Oklahoma College of Public Health, and the West Virginia University School of Medicine.

Karen Goldsteen, PhD, is Research Associate Professor in the Graduate Program in Public Health at SUNY, Stony Brook. She received an MPH from the Columbia University School of Public Health and a PhD in community health from the University of Illinois at Urbana-Champaign. She was a Pew Health Policy Fellow at the University of California, San Francisco.

David G. Graham, MD, MPH, is the former Chief Deputy Commissioner and Director of Public Health of the Suffolk County Department of Health Services. As the Director of Public Health, he managed epidemiology and disease control, public health protection, bioterrorism preparedness, preventive services, and the arthropodborne disease laboratory. As Chief Deputy Commissioner, he managed several major divisions, including public health, patient care, community mental hygiene, services for children with special needs, environmental quality, emergency medical services, and forensic sciences. His career in public health spans nearly 30 years.

Introduction to Public Health

Raymond L. Goldsteen, DrPH
Karen Goldsteen, PhD
David G. Graham, MD, MPH

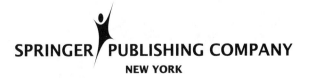
SPRINGER PUBLISHING COMPANY
NEW YORK

Springer Publishing Company, LLC
11 West 42nd Street
New York, NY 10036
www.springerpub.com

Acquisitions Editor: Jennifer Perillo
Senior Production Editor: Diane Davis
Cover Design: Joseph De Pinho
Composition: Absolute Service, Inc.; Project Manager, Pablo Apostol

ISBN: 978-0-8261-4152-1
E-book ISBN: 978-0-8261-4153-8

10 11 12 13/ 5 4 3 2 1

The author and the publisher of this Work have made every effort to use sources believed to be reliable to provide information that is accurate and compatible with the standards generally accepted at the time of publication. Because medical science is continually advancing, our knowledge base continues to expand. Therefore, as new information becomes available, changes in procedures become necessary. We recommend that the reader always consult current research and specific institutional policies before performing any clinical procedure. The author and publisher shall not be liable for any special, consequential, or exemplary damages resulting, in whole or in part, from the readers' use of, or reliance on, the information contained in this book. The publisher has no responsibility for the persistence or accuracy of URLs for external or third-party Internet Web sites referred to in this publication and does not guarantee that any content on such Web sites is, or will remain, accurate or appropriate.

Library of Congress Cataloging-in-Publication Data

Goldsteen, Raymond L.
  Introduction to public health / Raymond L. Goldsteen, Karen Goldsteen, David G. Graham.
     p. ; cm.
  Includes bibliographical references and index.
  ISBN 978-0-8261-4152-1 (alk. paper) — ISBN 978-0-8261-4153-8 (e-book)   .
  1. Public health. I. Goldsteen, Karen. II. Graham, David (David G.) III. Title.
  [DNLM: 1. Public Health Practice. WA 100]
  RA425.G58 2010
  362.1—dc22
                                    2010043653

Printed in the United States of America by Bang Printing.

This book is dedicated to public health professionals everywhere, who care deeply about the people they serve and strive daily to make the conditions in which they live healthful.

Contents

Preface

Public health is the ultimate"big tent." How do we introduce such a vast and glorious field to the uninitiated? How do we interest them in becoming public health professionals themselves, who will then offer their skills and enthusiasm in service of public health goals? As lifelong public health professionals who have taught public health to undergraduate and graduate students for many years, this was our aim in writing an Introduction to Public Health.

There is an urgent need to develop the public health perspective in more people to deal with the wide ranging problems that threaten health today. Despite many improvements in health and the conditions that promote health in recent years, there are areas of deep concern. These include the deterioration of global water supplies; stress on world food supplies and the resulting hunger suffered by millions daily; warming of the earth and its adverse impact on the natural environment; manmade catastrophes related to industrialization that expose people needlessly to toxins and injury; wars that leave millions homeless and without adequate food, water, and shelter and a stable social environment in which to live and raise children; and disparities in access to resources needed to promote health and well-being. For the many in the United States, these troubles may seem far away—difficulties that happen only in other countries and parts of the world—but they either exist here or have an impact on us indirectly.

These problems are amplified in the United States by the current breakdown in civic discourse and the polarization of people and politicians along cultural, political, educational, racial, and economic lines. The conditions that helped us to become a great nation—tolerance of diversity and access to opportunity regardless of race, religion, social status, or family heritage—are threatened. Social justice is under attack. Economic injustice is on the rise.

Yet, public health offers an antidote. We have a proud history of fighting for social justice and the conditions needed for health: Clean water; a safe and nutritious food supply; adequate sewage and garbage disposal; safe housing and workplaces; and infectious disease control. These are just a few of the areas of health improvement that public health has pioneered. We have a bold mission that gives direction and meaning to our practice. We have supported and helped provide women's suffrage, civil rights, reproductive rights, and access to medical care for seniors and the poor through Medicaid and Medicare. We have established premier organizations such as the Centers for Disease Control and Prevention and the World Health Organization, which advocate, monitor, and intervene to improve health and well-being for all people.

This volume makes no attempt to be a comprehensive description of public health. It was written to provide a framework for understanding this complex field. Further enrichment in the classroom and through assignments and exercises will be needed to fill-in the picture. Our hope is that it will be used to inform those seeking their professional identity and purpose about the values, goals, achievements, practice, and especially promise of public health in the hope that they will join us in working to fulfill that promise as future practitioners of public health. We need new leaders who will take up the mantle of such heroes of epidemiology and staunch advocates of public health as John Snow, Lemuel Shattuck, Joseph Goldberger, and Jack Geiger and face the challenges of improving the public's health and increasing social justice with courage, vision, and commitment.

We wish to acknowledge the help of our wonderful students Skye Ostreicher, Chris Gladwin, Dennis Dorf, and Luxi Ji.

Introduction to Public Health

1

Introduction and Overview

THE PROMISE OF PUBLIC HEALTH

Every year since 1873, the American Public Health Association (APHA) has held an annual meeting—a huge event attended by thousands of people, containing hundreds of sessions, over a period of nearly a week. The meeting expresses the public health priorities for that year and gives forum to the full range of current public health issues and activities. Current scientific and educational programs represent all sections, special interest groups, and caucuses. In the 2009 APHA annual meeting in Philadelphia, a typical recent year, the 27 sections, 6 special primary interest groups (SPIGs), and 17 caucuses were represented.

Among the sections were the following:

- Alcohol, Tobacco, and Other Drugs;
- Chiropractic Health Care;
- Community Health Planning and Policy Development;
- International Health;
- Maternal and Child Health;
- Medical Care;
- Mental Health;
- Occupational Health and Safety;
- Oral Health;
- Podiatric Health;
- Population, Reproductive and Sexual Health;
- Statistics; and
- Vision Care.

The caucuses included caucus on the following:

- Homelessness;
- Public Health and the Faith Community;
- Refugee and Immigrant Health;

1

- Community-Based Public Health; and
- Health Equity and Public Hospitals Caucus.

The six SPIGs were the following:

- Alternative and Complementary Health Practices;
- Community Health Workers;
- Ethics;
- Health Informatics Information Technology;
- Health Law; and
- Veterinary Public Health.

The theme of the 2009 APHA Annual Meeting was *Water and Public Health*, and sessions directly related to this issue included:

- Water, development, and human rights;
- Water, women, and maternal mortality; and
- Drinking water: source-to-tap public health aspects.

However, a sampling of other session titles includes:

- Assessment of Static Standing Exposures Among Manufacturing Workers;
- Dating and Intimate Partner Violence;
- Climate Changes, Migration, and Its Impact on Health;
- Teaching Human Genetics in Classrooms to Increase Students' Health Literacy;
- Pounding the Pavement Together: Lessons Learned From an Environmental Assessment of East Harlem;
- Promoting Postdisaster Resilience and Mental Health Through Community Capacity Building in New Orleans;
- A Decade on the Mean Streets: A New Typology for Understanding Health Choices of Those Living in Poverty;
- Creating Community Advocates Using a Critical Health Literacy Model;
- Portable Farmer's Market: Mobile Vending to Promote Healthy Food Access in Vulnerable Communities;
- Purchasing Healthy Foods in Restricted Built Environments;
- Barriers to Physical Activity Among Adolescents With Mobility Disabilities;
- Eat, Drink, and Deplete? Long-Term Threats to Health, Environment, and Food Systems;

- Reimbursement for Rehabilitation Services for Older Individuals Who Are Blind: Improving Cost-Effectiveness and Satisfaction;
- Preparing for Threats of Legal Challenges to Public Health Laws;
- An Initiative to Apply Health Protection Mechanisms in International Trade Regulations;
- Digital Disparities: The Role of Technology/HIT in the Development and Elimination of Health Disparities;
- Health Care Reform;
- Reforming Access to Dental Care; and
- Overview of the Public Health Approach to Youth Suicide Prevention.

This small sample of topics at one meeting indicates the diversity and abundance of subjects that concern public health professionals.

In reviewing the topics from the APHA Annual Meeting in 2009 and noting their scope and variety, we may be motivated to ask, "What does teaching human genetics have in common with purchasing healthy foods?" "What is the link between international trade regulations and youth suicide prevention?" "How are climate change and community capacity building connected?" "What is the link between intimate partner violence and drinking water?" Similarly, when we examine the composition of the public health workforce through job postings at the APHA Annual Meeting and other public health employment sites, we see positions as different as sanitarian, community organizer, health educator, environmental safety specialist, infectious disease manager, epidemiologist, microbiologist, data analyst, and reproductive health specialist. Again, we may ask, "What is the common thread that connects these disparate types of employment?"

The answer to these questions lies in the following statement written in 1988 by the Institute of Medicine's Committee for the Study of the Future of Public Health:

The broad mission of public health is to "fulfill society's interest in assuring conditions in which people can be healthy." p. 1

This statement was intended to capture the essence of the historical and present work of public health, and it binds us together by identifying our common bond. It asserts that we, in the field of public health, are engaged in a great societal endeavor to create the circumstances that make health possible. We may have little in common on a day-to-day basis with our fellow public health professionals, and our knowledge base and skills may vary widely from others in our field. However, our mission is the same, and each of us contributes to that mission in some important way, which we will begin to explicate in the coming pages. Before proceeding, though, we need to examine this statement more closely to understand its assumptions and implications. By examining these, we understand our commonalities with other professionals focused on health—particularly the clinical professions such as medicine, nursing, dentistry, physical therapy, and others—as well as our unique role among health professionals.

First, the idea of assuring health for all people—the entire population— is embedded in the mission statement. Although public health will focus on different populations within the larger population when planning services, we are obligated to ensure health-producing conditions for all people—not just the poor, not just the rich, but people of all incomes; not only the young or the old, but people of all ages; not exclusively Whites or Blacks, but people of all races and ethnicities.

Second, the belief that a society benefits from having a healthy populace is clear in the public health mission's phrase "to fulfill society's interest . . ." The work of public health is a societal effort with a societal benefit. Public health takes the view held by many professions and societies throughout human history that healthy people are more productive and creative, and these attributes create a strong society. Healthy people lead to better societies. For the welfare of the society, as a whole, it is better for people to be healthy than sick. There will be less dependence, less lost time from productive work, and a greater pool of productive workers, soldiers, parents, and others needed to accomplish society's goals. Thus, as public health professionals, we believe that society has an interest in the health of the population; it benefits the society, as a whole, when people are healthy.

Third, the public health mission acknowledges that health is not guaranteed. The mission states that "people *can* (not *will*) be healthy." Health is a possibility, although we intend through our actions to make it highly probable. However, not everyone will be healthy even if each one exists in health-producing conditions. Public health efforts will not result in every person being healthy—although we certainly would not object to that kind of success. Rather, public health creates conditions in which people can be healthy. Whether any single individual is healthy, we acknowledge, will vary.

The fourth and fifth assumptions differentiate public health from the healing, or clinical, professions—medicine, nursing, dentistry, physical therapy, physician assistant, and others—that we will refer to for simplicity throughout the remainder of this book as the clinical professions. All clinical professions believe in the obligation of their practitioners to care for all people in need of their services. Further, they accept the fallibility of their professions; not every patient will be "cured" regardless of the effort expended by the practitioner to bring about this outcome. Finally, all health care professions believe that improving health is a benefit, not only to the individuals treated, but also to the society, as a whole. These beliefs, for example, are evident in the widely referenced Physician's Oath adopted by the World Medical Association Declaration of Geneva (1948 and amended by the 22nd World Medical Assembly in 1968):

At the time of being admitted as a member of the medical professions:

- I solemnly pledge myself to consecrate my life to the service of humanity;
- I will give to my teachers the respect and gratitude which is their due;
- I will practice my profession with conscience and dignity; the health of my patient will be my first consideration;
- I will maintain by all the means in my power, the honor and the noble traditions of the medical profession; my colleagues will be my brothers;
- I will not permit considerations of religion, nationality, race, party politics or social standing to intervene between my duty and my patient;
- I will maintain the utmost respect for human life from the time of conception, even under threat, I will not use my medical knowledge contrary to the laws of humanity;
- I make these promises solemnly, freely and upon my honor. (*Declaration of Geneva* [1948]. Adopted by the General Assembly of World Medical Association at Geneva Switzerland, September 1948.)

Thus, public health shares with the clinical professions a fundamental caring for humanity through concern for health. For these reasons, public health is sometimes viewed as a type of clinical profession.

Prevention: The Cornerstone of Public Health

However, if we examine the public health mission closely, we find that public health is complementary to the clinical professions, but not subsumed by it. The critical differences between public health and the clinical professions relate to their strategies for creating a healthy populace. The fourth and fifth assumptions embedded in the public health mission are that prevention is the preferred strategy and to be successful, prevention must address the "conditions," that is, environment in the fullest sense, in which people live. The classic and defining public health strategy is to prevent poor health by "assuring conditions in which people can be healthy."

This choice of a prevention and environment-based strategy clearly distinguishes public health from the clinical professions, which focus on diagnosing individuals and treating them when they have health problems detectable by clinical methods—history, physical examinations, laboratory tests, imaging, and so forth. Here, an understanding of the different types of prevention—primary, secondary, and tertiary—is necessary to distinguish between public health and the clinical professions.

Primary, Secondary, and Tertiary Prevention

There are three types of prevention: primary, secondary, and tertiary. Fos and Fine (2000) define primary, secondary, and tertiary prevention as follows:

> Primary prevention is concerned with eliminating risk factors for a disease. Secondary prevention focuses on early detection and treatment of disease (subclinical and clinical). Tertiary prevention attempts to eliminate or moderate disability associated with advanced disease. (pp. 108–109)

Primary prevention intends to prevent the development of disease and the occurrence of injury, and thus, to reduce their incidence in the population. Examples of primary prevention include the use of automobile seat belts, condom use, skin protection from ultraviolet light, and tobacco-use cessation programs. Secondary prevention is concerned with treating disease after it has developed so that there are no permanent adverse consequences; early detection is emphasized. Secondary prevention activities are intended to identify the existence of disease early so that treatments that might not be as effective when applied later can be of benefit. Tertiary prevention focuses on the optimum treatment of clinically apparent and clearly identified disease to reduce complications to the greatest possible degree. Tertiary prevention often involves limiting disability that occurs if disease and injury are not effectively treated.

The central focus of clinical professions is to restore health or prevent exacerbation of health problems. Thus, health care is primarily concerned with secondary and tertiary prevention: (a) early detection, diagnosis, and treatment of conditions that can be cured or reversed (secondary prevention); and (b) treatment of chronic diseases and other conditions to prevent exacerbation and minimize future complications (tertiary prevention). The health care system undoubtedly has its smallest impact on primary prevention, once again that group of interventions that focus on preventing disease, illness, and injury from occurring. Moreover, as Evans and Stoddart (1994) argue, other than for immunization, the major focus of the health care system's primary prevention activities is on the behavioral determinants of health, rather than structural or policy factors:

> The focus on individual risk factors and specific diseases has tended to lead not away from but back to the health care system itself. Interventions, particularly those addressing personal life-styles, are offered in the form of "provider counseling" for smoking cessation, seatbelt use, or dietary modification. These in turn are subsumed under a more general and rapidly growing set of interventions attempting to modify risk factors through transactions between clinicians and individual patients.
>
> The "product line" of the health care system is thus extended to deal with a more broadly defined set of "diseases": unhealthy behaviors. The boundary becomes blurred between, e.g., heart disease as manifest in symptoms, or in elevated serum cholesterol measurements, or in excessive consumption of fats. All are "diseases" and represent a "need" for health care intervention. . . . The behaviors of large and powerful organizations, or the effects of economic and social policies, public and private, [are] not brought under scrutiny. (pp. 43–44)

Another often-quoted modern version of the Hippocratic Oath written by Louis Lasagna (1970) in *The Doctors' Dilemmas* provides an example of the difference between the clinical professional, whose improvement strategy is based on diagnosis and treatment of individuals.

I swear to fulfill, to the best of my ability and judgment, this covenant:

- I will respect the hard-won scientific gains of those physicians in whose steps I walk, and gladly share such knowledge as is mine with those who are to follow.
- I will apply, for the benefit of the sick, all measures [that] are required, avoiding those twin traps of overtreatment and therapeutic nihilism.
- I will remember that there is art to medicine as well as science, and that warmth, sympathy, and understanding may outweigh the surgeon's knife or the chemist's drug.
- I will not be ashamed to say "I know not," nor will I fail to call in my colleagues when the skills of another are needed for a patient's recovery.
- I will respect the privacy of my patients, for their problems are not disclosed to me that the world may know. Most especially must I tread with care in matters of life and death. If it is given me to save a life, all thanks. But it may also be within my power to take a life; this awesome responsibility must be faced with great humbleness and awareness of my own frailty. Above all, I must not play at God.
- I will remember that I do not treat a fever chart, a cancerous growth, but a sick human being, whose illness may affect the person's family and economic stability. My responsibility includes these related problems, if I am to care adequately for the sick.
- I will prevent disease whenever I can, for prevention is preferable to cure.
- I will remember that I remain a member of society, with special obligations to all my fellow human beings, those sound of mind and body as well as the infirm.
- If I do not violate this oath, may I enjoy life and art, respected while I live and remembered with affection thereafter. May I always act so as to preserve the finest traditions of my calling and may I long experience the joy of healing those who seek my help.

Although it contains one statement about the importance of primary prevention—"I will prevent disease whenever I can"—it is clear that the physician is viewed as a healer of individuals. The idea conveyed by this statement is that the physician uses clinical tools to treat health problems that have already begun, which is very different from the public health professional whose main goal is primary prevention of health problems employing strategies based on improving the circumstances in which people live.

Secondary and Tertiary Prevention and Public Health

The public health emphasis on primary prevention does not mean that public health has no role or interest in secondary and tertiary prevention. On the contrary, public health professionals are vitally interested and involved in secondary and tertiary prevention. However, their focus is on ensuring access to effective clinical care, rather than on providing the care itself. Preventing long-term consequences of health problems and limiting the progression of illness, disability, and disease is dependent on access to excellent medical care. Thus, ensuring that all people have health insurance has been an important issue for public health in the United States, as has health care reform that improves the quality and efficiency of health care. Access to primary care and the specialties has historically been a target of public health initiatives. Other issues that impact on people's ability to access and use health care appropriately are important, as well. These include such concerns as transportation to health providers, cultural competence of health care providers, health literacy of patients, and efficiency and effectiveness of health care delivery.

An example of public health's interest in secondary and tertiary prevention is the development of Medically Underserved Areas (MUAs), Medically Underserved Populations (MUPs), and Health Professional Shortage Areas (HPSAs):

Medically Underserved Areas/Populations are areas or populations designated by HRSA as having: too few primary care providers, high infant mortality, high poverty and/or high elderly population. Health Professional Shortage Areas (HPSAs) are designated by HRSA as having shortages of primary medical care, dental or mental health providers and may be geographic (a county or service area), demographic (low income population), or institutional (comprehensive health center, federally qualified health center or other public facility). (U.S. Department of Health and Human Services [DHHS], 2010)

Through designation of areas and populations as medically underserved, programs responding to their medical needs have been developed. These programs address the concerns about access to quality medical care in specific populations and geographic areas, which is necessary for secondary and tertiary prevention. Public health is vitally interested and involved in the identification of MUPs and MUAs, as well as in the development of programs to meet these needs.

If we were to apply the language of the clinical professions to public health, we might say that classic public health "diagnoses" and "treats" the circumstances in which people live and the success of public health is measured by the health of the populations living in the "treated" circumstances. However, the language of epidemiology and ecology are preferred to describe the work of public health professionals, as we will explore later in this chapter. In summary, public health is proactive, rather than curative: Do not wait until people get sick and then treat them. Rather, go out and create conditions that promote health and prevent disease, injury, and disability.

An infectious disease outbreak provides an example of the complementary roles played by public health and clinical professionals:

In early December 2009, CDC's PulseNet staff identified a multistate cluster of 14 *E. coli* O157:H7 isolates with a particular DNA fingerprint or pulsed-field gel electrophoresis (PFGE) pattern reported from 13 states. CDC's OutbreakNet team began working with state and local partners to gather epidemiologic information about persons in the cluster to determine if any of the ill individuals had been exposed to the same food source(s). Health officials in several states who were investigating reports of *E. coli* O157:H7 illnesses in this cluster found that most ill persons had consumed beef, many in restaurants. CDC is continuing to collaborate with state and local health departments in an attempt to gather additional epidemiologic information and share this information with FSIS. At this time, at least some of the illnesses appear to be associated with products subject to a recent FSIS recall. (Centers for Disease Control and Prevention [CDC], 2010a)

Thus, public health officials collaborated with physicians, who had diagnosed and treated patients with the disease, as well as with officials from the U.S. Department of Agriculture's Food Safety and Inspection Service to determine the source of the infection and how to prevent reoccurrence of infection in other people. Public health officials addressed the circumstances in which the infection developed so that others would be spared the illness resulting from exposure to the pathogen.

Summary

The control of an infectious disease outbreak is an example of the promise of public health—collective action that prevents the occurrence of disease, disability, and premature death by "assuring conditions in which people can be healthy." Because of public health, people will have the opportunity, to the best of our knowledge and capabilities, to be healthy. Public health, as a field and as a collection of practicing professionals, will ensure that the environment in which people lead their lives promotes health.

Underlying this mission is a commitment to social justice because it assumes that all people are deserving of healthy conditions in which to live— not just the rich, but people of all incomes; not only the young or the old, but people of all ages; not exclusively the majority race or ethnicity, but people of all races and ethnicities. Public health is a leader and plays an integral role in carrying out this societal obligation. For this reason, public health is often associated with advocating and providing services for the structurally disadvantaged—those with the least power in their social circumstances. As Krieger and Birn (1998) argue powerfully:

Social justice is the foundation of public health. This powerful proposition—still contested-first emerged around 150 years ago during the formative years of public health as both a modern movement and a profession. It is an assertion that reminds us that public health is indeed a public matter, that societal patterns of disease and death, of health and well-being, of bodily integrity and disintegration, intimately reflect the workings of the body politic for good and for ill. It is a statement that asks us, pointedly, to remember that worldwide dramatic declines—and continued inequalities- in mortality and morbidity signal as much the victories and defeats of social movements to create a just, fair, caring, and inclusive world as they do the achievements and unresolved challenges of scientific research and technology. To declare that social justice is the foundation of public health is to call upon and nurture that invincible human spirit that led so many of us to enter the field of public health in the first place: a spirit that has a compelling desire to make the world a better place, free of misery, inequity, and preventable suffering, a world in which we all can live, love, work, play, ail and die with our dignity intact and our humanity cherished. (p. 1603)

The cornerstone of public health is prevention, particularly primary prevention. Prevention is public health's historic and ideal approach to promoting health, and the distinguishing public health prevention strategy is to influence the "conditions" (i.e., the environment, in the fullest sense) in which people live. The classic and defining public health strategy to prevent poor health is to assure "conditions in which people can be healthy." A commitment to social justice underlies the public health mission to achieve health-promoting conditions for all. How public health has attempted to ensure conditions that promote health is the story of the practice of public health, which we will introduce next.

THE PRACTICE OF PUBLIC HEALTH

What is entailed in "assuring conditions in which people can be healthy"? In the answer to this question lies the source of the varied interests, knowledge, and skills that differentiate public health professionals from each other. The causes of poor health are many and complex, and therefore, solutions are complex and diverse, as well. Public health conceptualizes and organizes this complexity by applying the concepts and principles of ecology, which views individuals as embedded within their environment, or context. The ecological approach to understanding how health is either fostered or undermined is fundamental to public health practice.

However, before we can discuss the practice of public health, that is, the ways that public health professionals attempt to influence context and promote health, we will discuss how we define health and conceptualize the complex set of factors that affect health, called the determinants of health.

How Do We Define Health?

The most famous and influential definition of health is the one developed by the World Health Organization (WHO) in the 1940s: "Health is a state of complete physical, mental and social well being and not merely, the absence of disease or infirmity." It was adopted in 1946 and has not been amended since 1948 (WHO, 1946). Many subsequent definitions have taken an equally broad view of health, including that of the International Epidemiological Association: A state characterized by anatomical, physiological and psychological integrity, ability to perform personally valued family, work, and community roles; ability to deal with physical, biological, psychological, and social stress; a feeling of well-being; and freedom from the risk of disease and untimely death.

Both definitions exemplify the tendency over the second half of the 20th century to enlarge the definition of health beyond morbidity, disability, and premature mortality to include sense of well-being, ability to adapt to change, and social functioning. However, in practice, the more limited view of health as diagnosable morbidity, mortality, and disability usually guides public health efforts to improve health status. As Young (1998) writes, "Indeed, the WHO definition is 'honored in repetition, rarely in application.' Health may become so inclusive that virtually all human endeavors, including the pursuit of happiness, are considered within its domain" (p. 2). In this book, as in general public health practice, the term *health* will refer to the more restricted definition—diagnosable morbidity, disability, and premature mortality.

The Determinants of Health

There are many influences on individual and population health. As the WHO (2010) puts it:

> Many factors combine together to affect the health of individuals and communities. Whether people are healthy or not, is determined by their circumstances and environment. To a large extent, factors such as where we live, the state of our environment, genetics, our income and education level, and our relationships with friends and family all have considerable impacts on health, whereas the more commonly considered factors such as access and use of health care services often have less of an impact.

It is generally accepted that the determinants of health include the physical environment—natural and built—and the social environment, as well as individual behavior, genetic inheritance, and health care (Evans & Stoddart, 1994). Note that although we talk about the "determinants of health," they are usually discussed in terms of how they relate to poor health—the determinants of poor health. A brief overview of the determinants of health follows.

Physical Environment

Physical environment includes both the natural and built environments. The natural environment is defined by the features of an area that include its topography, weather, soil, water, animal life, and other such attributes; and the built environment is defined by the structures that people have created for housing, commerce, transportation, government, recreation, and so forth. Health threats arise from both the physical and built environments. Common health threats related to the natural environment include weather-related disasters such as tornados, hurricanes, and earthquakes, as well as exposure to infectious disease agents that are endemic in a region such as *Plasmodium falciparum*, the microbe that causes malaria and is endemic in Africa.

Health threats related to the built environment include exposure to toxins and unsafe conditions, particularly in occupational and residential settings where people spend most of their time. Many occupations expose workers to disease-causing substances, high risk of injury, and other physical risks. For example, the greatest health threats to U.S. farm workers are injuries from farm machinery and falls that result in sprains, strains, fractures, and abrasions (Myers, 2001). There are well-documented health threats to office workers from indoor air pollution, found by research beginning in the 1970s, including passive exposure to tobacco smoke, nitrogen dioxide from gas-fueled cooking stoves, formaldehyde exposure, "radon daughter" exposure, and other health problems encountered in sealed office buildings (Samet, Marbury, & Spengler, 1987; U.S. Environmental Protection Agency, 2006). In residential settings, exposure to pollutants from nearby industrial facilities, power plants, toxic waste sites, or a high volume of traffic presents hazards for many. In the United States, these threats are increasingly known to have a disproportionately heavy impact on low-income and minority communities (CDC, 2003; Institute of Medicine, 1999).

Social Environment

The social environment is defined by the major organizing concepts of human life: society, community, religion, social network, family, and occupation. Individuals' lives are governed by religious, political, economic, and organizational rules—formal and informal—that reflect the cultural norms, values, and beliefs of their particular social context. These formal and informal rules, and the values, beliefs and norms they reflect, have historical roots, and they affect how individuals live and behave; their relationships with others; and what resources and opportunities individuals have to influence their lives. They shape the relationship between individuals and the natural environment and how the built environment is conceived and developed.

An important aspect of the social environment is the status, resources, and power that individuals have within their social environment or context. In the United States and other Western countries, this aspect is indicated by an individual's socioeconomic status—a combination of education, occupation, and income/wealth—and an individual's race and/or ethnicity. Socioeconomic status is associated with significant variations in health status and risk for health problems. There is a large literature demonstrating the relationship between socioeconomic status and health, including a gradient in which the higher the socioeconomic status, the better the health (Lynch, Smith, Kaplan, & House, 2000). The famous Whitehall Study of English civil servants in the 1970s was one of the first and most influential to demonstrate this relationship:

> The Whitehall Study consists of a group of people of relatively uniform ethnic background, all employed in stable office-based jobs and not subject to industrial hazards, unemployment, or extremes of poverty or affluence; all live and work in Greater London and adjoining areas. Yet in this relative homogeneous population, we observed a gradient in mortality— each group experiencing a higher mortality than the one above it in the hierarchy. The difference in mortality between the highest and lowest grades was threefold. (Marmot, Bobak, & Smith, 1995, p. 173)

Similarly, much research indicates that disparities in health status exist between racial and ethnic minority groups. Minority Americans including African Americans, Hispanic/Latinos, Native Americans, and Pacific Islanders generally have poorer health outcomes than do Whites. The preventable and treatable conditions for which disparities between majority and minority Americans have been shown include cardiovascular disease, diabetes, asthma, cancer, and HIV/AIDS (DHHS, 1998). Although race and ethnicity do not "explain" these disparities, they point to the need for explanations. Discrimination and its consequences are a recent focus for investigations attempting to explain racial and ethnic disparities (Krieger, 2000; Mays, Cochran, & Barnes, 2007).

Nonphysical occupational factors also affect health. For example, a great deal of research demonstrates the relationship between poor health outcomes and the psychosocial work environment. The demand–control model is one well-known theory, hypothesizing that employees with the highest psychological demands and the lowest decision-making latitude are at the highest risk for poor health outcomes (Karasek, Baker, Marxer, Ahlbom, & Theorell, 1981; Karasek et al., 1998; Theorell, 2000). In addition, job loss and threat of job loss also have a negative impact on health. Evidence suggests that transitions from employment to unemployment adversely affect physical health and psychological well-being among working-age persons (Dooley, Fielding, & Levi, 1996; Kasl & Jones, 2000; Kasl, Rodriguez, & Lasch, 1998).

Another large body of research on the social environment and health focuses on social integration, social networks, and social support (Berkman & Glass, 2000). For example, numerous studies over the past 20 years have found that people who are isolated or disengaged from others have a higher risk of premature death. In addition, research has found that survival of cardiovascular disease events and stroke is higher among people with close ties to others, particularly emotional ties. Social relations have been found to predict compliance with medical care recommendations, adaptation to adverse life events such as death of a loved one or natural disaster, and coping with long-term difficulties such as caring for a dependent parent or a disabled child.

A great deal of research in the area of social support was conducted during the 1960s and 1970s. A seminal review article published in 1977 by Kaplan, Cassel, and Gore identified methodological issues that needed to be addressed. Since then, there has been further specification of the relationship between social support and health to explain the relationship. For example, Cohen (2004) discusses three factors that indicate different aspects of social relationships: social integration, negative interaction, and social support, each influencing health through different mechanisms. Thoits (1982) reanalyzed data to test the hypothesis that disadvantaged sociodemographic groups such as low-income women are more vulnerable to the effects of life events because they experience more negative events and have fewer psychological resources to copy with them. Although the relationship between social support and health is still not well understood, it is found over and over again in health studies.

Genetic Inheritance

Our knowledge about the effects of genetic inheritance on health is growing rapidly. It is understood that, with few exceptions, disease processes "are determined both by environmental and by genetic factors. These usually interact, and individuals with a particular set of genes may be either more or less likely, if exposed, to be at risk of developing a particular disease. These effects can be measured by showing that the relative risk of exposure to an environmental factor is significantly greater (or lesser) for the subgroup with the abnormal gene, than the risk in those without" (Pencheon, Guest, Melzer, & Gray, 2001, p. 544).

Health Behavior

The term *health behavior* can refer to behaviors that are beneficial to health. However, the term is generally used in the negative to refer to behaviors that harm health, including smoking, abusing alcohol or other substances, failing to use seat belts or practicing other unsafe behaviors, making unhealthy food choices, and not engaging in adequate physical activity.

The effect of health behaviors on health status has been widely studied and found to be an important determinant of health. Consider the 10 leading causes of death, as of 2006, as characterized by diagnosed disease or condition in the general population: diseases of the heart, malignant neoplasms (cancer), cerebrovascular diseases (stroke), chronic lower respiratory diseases, unintentional injuries (accidents), diabetes mellitus, Alzheimer's disease, influenza and pneumonia, nephritis, nephrotic syndrome and nephrosis, and septicemia. The next five leading causes of death were intentional self-harm (suicide), chronic liver disease and cirrhosis, essential hypertension and hypertensive renal disease, Parkinson's disease, and assault (homicide) (Centers for Disease Control and Prevention, 2010b). In one way or another, personal health behavior has an impact on the occurrence in any given individual of most of the diseases and conditions on this list. Further, looking at the cause of death in a different way, that is, by major contributing cause of the disease to which the death was attributed rather than by the disease itself, in the first study of its kind, McGinnis and Foege (1993) showed that, as of 1990, the leading factors were tobacco use, dietary patterns, sedentary lifestyle, alcohol consumption, microbial agents, toxic agents, firearms, sexual behavior, motor vehicles, and use of illicit drugs. As of 2002, the situation remained the same (McGinnis, Williams-Russo, & Knickman, 2002).

Health Care as a Determinant of Health

If we argue that health is the product of multiple factors including genetic inheritance, the physical environment, and the social environment, as well as an individual's behavioral and biologic response to these factors, we see that health care has an impact late in the causal chain leading to disease, illness, and injury. Often by the time the individual interacts with the health care system, the determinants of health have had their impact on their health status, for better or for worse. Thus, the need for health care may be seen as a failure to prevent the determinants of health from adversely affecting the individual patient.

The success of any health care system is affected by the other determinants of health. Genetic predisposition to breast cancer may limit the long-term success rates of cancer treatment. Continued exposure to toxins in the environment or at work may decrease the likelihood that the physician can stabilize an individual with allergies. Health behaviors, such as smoking or substance abuse, may stymie the best health care system when treating an individual with lung disease. The lack of support at home for changes in behaviors or adherence to medical regimens may undermine the ability of the health care system to treat an individual with diabetes successfully. Poverty, race, and ethnicity often limit access to health care, and therefore, the ability of physicians to diagnose and treat health problems effectively (Smedley, Stith, & Nelson, 2003). We recognize that health, as well as health care, exist within a biological, physical, and social context, and all of these factors influence the level of probability of success of a health care system. Health care is only one determinant of health.

Relationship Between the Determinants of Health

The determinants of health do not act independently of each other. They are interconnected, and the concepts of ecology provide the framework for understanding how to model their interconnectedness. In the most general sense, the ecological approach means that the person is viewed as embedded in the environment—both social and physical—and is both influenced by and influences that environment. Stokols (1996) outlines the history of ecology, and social ecology, which are fundamental to the public health perspective and its practice:

> The term ecology refers to the study of the relationships between organisms and their environments. Early ecological analyses of the relations between plant and animal populations and their natural habitats were later extended and applied to the study of human communities and environments within the fields of sociology, psychology, and public health. The field of social ecology, which emerged during the mid 1960s and early 1970s, gives greater attention to the social, institutional, and cultural contexts of people-environment relations than did earlier versions of human ecology, which focused primarily on biologic processes and the geographic environment. (p. 285)

Stokols (1996) identifies core principles of social ecology that make it an appropriate overarching paradigm for public health. First, ecological models may include all aspects of the environment that impact health including physical, social, and cultural aspects. Second, ecological models include characteristics of individuals, and for example, can incorporate their genetic heritage, psychological attributes, and behavioral practices. Third, concepts from systems theory are used to understand the interplay between environmental and individual characteristics and their mutual influence on health.

> For instance, people-environment transactions are characterized by cycles of mutual influence, in which the physical and social features of settings directly influence occupants' health and, concurrently, the participants in settings modify the healthfulness of their surroundings through their individual and collective actions. (p. 286)

Fourth, the ecological perspective emphasizes the interdependence of all factors contributing to health including the nearby and distant factors, as well as those in different domains such as family, work, neighborhood, and community.

> Thus, efforts to promote human health must take into account the inter-dependencies that exist among immediate and more distant environments (e.g., the "spill-over" of workplace and commuting stress to residential environments; and the influence of state and national ordinances on the healthfulness of occupational settings. (Stokols, 1996, p. 286)

Fifth, the ecological perspective is interdisciplinary, which is required for public health practice. With the multitude of factors that affect human health, many disciplines are required to understand the interplay between them and their effect on health and to bring about health improvement. "Thus, ecologically based health research incorporates multiple levels of analysis and diverse methodologies . . . for assessing the healthfulness of settings and the well-being of persons and groups" (Stokols, 1996, p. 286).

The classic 1959 book, *Mirage of Health*, by Rene Dubos provides an example of how the ecological approach is applied to human health. Dubos describes the causes of the tuberculosis epidemic in the tenements of 1900 New York City and other U.S. cities. He recounts

> The story of the roundabout way in which a microscopic fungus prob-ably native to Central America destroyed the potato crop in Ireland and exerted thereby a dramatic influence on the destiny of the Irish people, illustrating the complexity of the interplay between the external environ-ment and the affairs of man. (pp. 96–97)

Dubos's description of the factors contributing to the development of the tuberculosis epidemic includes international exploration and trade by Europeans subsequent to the 15th century that transported a native plant, the wild potato, from the Andes to Ireland and elsewhere in Europe; the improvement of the wild potato in Europe for large yields, which made the plant more susceptible to infection than the wild varieties; a fungus that accompanied the potato to Europe and was benign until it was enabled by unusually wet weather conditions to proliferate and destroy the potato crop in 1845 and 1846 in Ireland; the growth of the Irish population from 3.5–8 million between 1700 and 1840; the dependence on the potato for sustenance among the burgeoning Irish population; the political and economic dependence of Ireland on England that resulted in the food shortage following the destruction of the 1845 and 1846 potato crops; the disaster that followed in which a million Irish died of starvation and many more became susceptible to disease; and finally the mass emigration from Ireland to the United States in the middle of the 19th century where the immigrants took up residence in the crowded and unhealthy conditions of the tenements of industrial cities along the Atlantic coast.

> The profound upheaval in their way of life made them ready victims to all sorts of infection. The sudden and dramatic increase of tuberculosis mortality in the Philadelphia, New York and Boston Areas around 1850 can be traced in large part to the Irish immigrants who settled in these cities at that time. (Dubos, 1959, p. 100)

Dubos's account included many determinants of health including aspects of the social environment, the physical environment, and individual behavior. Interestingly, he does not mention health care, or its absence, as a factor leading to the tuberculosis epidemic, but then there was little that medicine offered at that time for the treatment of tuberculosis. His analysis of events incorporated the "causes of causes," which were political, economic, and cultural. These included the impetus among Europeans to explore and trade that caused the transport of the wild potato from Central America to Europe; the application of scientific principles to farming that caused the improvement of the potato; the political and economic relationships between Ireland and England that caused the dependence of the Irish on the potato for food; and so forth. We understand the disease, not only in terms of immediate individual actions, for example, sanitary habits of the individuals with tuberculosis, but in terms of societal attributes that reach back into history and relate to political and economic events and policies of the times.

Dubos's account exemplifies the ecological approach to understanding the causes of poor health—in this case, tuberculosis—which is the foundation of the public health orientation. Dubos's account links the determinants of health in a causal chain that ends in illness, disability, and premature death in the tenements of 19th-century American cities.

Ecological Models and Public Health Practice

The environment, or context, influences the way people live and their health outcomes, for better or for worse. That is, context can have positive or negative impacts on the health of individuals.

As a field, public health attempts to maintain or create healthy contexts in which people live and prevent or dismantle unhealthy contexts—to promote health and reduce morbidity, disability, and premature mortality.

The way in which public health attempts to affect contexts is the story of public health practice, and public health practice reflects public health ecological models. However, the ecological models in use change over time to respond to the health problems predominant in their day and incorporate the knowledge, beliefs, values, and resources of that time and place.

For example, in times and places where infectious diseases are predominant, models reflect the issues required to understand their spread and control. A classic public health model that uses the ecological approach for understanding and preventing disease is the epidemiological triangle with its agent-host-environment triad. The epidemiological triangle (see Figure 1.1) was developed and is used to understand infectious disease transmission and to provide a model for preventing transmission, and thus, infectious disease outbreaks. The three points of the triangle are the agent, host, and environment. The agent is the microbial organism that causes the infectious disease—virus, bacteria, protozoa, or fungus; the host is the organism that harbors the agent; and the environmental aspects included in an epidemiological triangle are those factors that facilitate transmission of the agent to the host. These could be aspects of the natural environment, the built environment, or the social environment, including policies. Time is considered in the triangle as the period between exposure to the agent

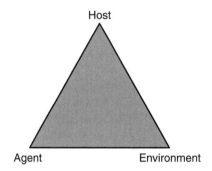

FIGURE 1.1   Epidemiological Triangle

and illness occurs; the period that it takes to recover from illness; or the period it takes an outbreak to subside. Prevention measures are those that disrupt the relationship between at least two of the factors in the triangle—agent, host, and environment.

Although there are no explicitly specified environmental factors included in the epidemiological triangle, the environment is central to conceptualizing disease transmission among individuals at risk (the hosts). The environment is the total of factors that enable the agent to infect the host. The environmental factors specified in the model can include, depending upon the disease itself, an array of social and physical attributes that permit the agent to infect the host. For example, Friis and Sellers (1996) write:

> The external environment is the sum total of influences that are not part of the host and comprises physical, climatologic, biologic, social, and economic components. The physical environment includes weather, temperature, humidity, geologic formations, and similar physical dimensions. Contrasted with the physical environment is the social environment, which is the totality of the behavioral, personality, attitudinal, and cultural characteristics of a group of people. Both these facets of the external environment have an impact on agents of disease and potential hosts because the environment may either enhance or diminish the survival of disease agents and may serve to bring agent and host into contact. (p. 315)

Because infectious diseases have a single agent, the epidemiological triangle works well as a model for understanding the development of these diseases. In the case of other kinds of diseases or health problems, it is not as helpful because of its emphasis on a single agent, its isolation of the agent from the environment, and its conceptually unspecified environment.

The wheel of causation is another model exemplifying the ecological approach (See Figure 1.2). It has also been used, but not as extensively as the epidemiological triangle for explaining infectious disease transmission. However, it has some advantages over the epidemiological triangle, as Peterson (1995) notes,

> Although it is not used as often as the epidemiological triangle model, it has several appealing attributes (Fig. 2). For instance, the wheel contains a hub with the host at its center. For our use, humans represent the host. Also, surrounding the host is the total environment divided into the biological, physical, and social environments. These divisions, of course, are not true divisions—there are considerable interactions among the environment types. Although it is a general model, the wheel of causation does illustrate the multiple etiological factors of human infectious diseases. (p. 147)

In general, every ecological model explaining the development of health (or poor health) contains a set of distal causes related to the environment—physical and/or social—and a set of proximal causes related to the individual—primarily behavioral. One of the major issues in developing public health models is where to place the emphasis and, thus, where to intervene to improve health? Is it at the individual level or at the environmental level? This issue is at the heart of public health practice.

Therefore, in the simplest conceptualization of prevention strategies, we have two choices: We can focus our efforts on changing individual behavior directly or on changing the environment in which individual behavior occurs. For example, after examining Dubos's description of the

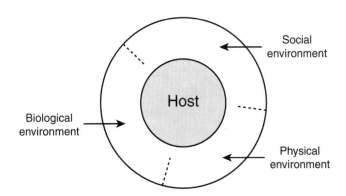

FIGURE 1.2   Wheel of Causation

development of the tuberculosis epidemics of the 1850s in the north-eastern cities of the United States, we might decide that tuberculosis should have been prevented by focusing on the sanitary habits of the Irish immigrants, which would have reduced the spread of disease from person to person. These habits might have included hand washing, housekeeping, food preparation practices, and so forth. Changing behavior might have taken the form of encouraging compliance through education or coercing compliance through surveillance and laws.

On the other hand, we might decide that the tuberculosis epidemics should have been prevented by changing the social, political, or physical environments. For instance, if the cities to which the Irish emigrated had provided more healthful housing and working conditions, the Irish immigrants would not have been as susceptible to illness, including tuberculosis. We might have targeted the crowding and other relevant conditions in the neighborhoods where the immigrants came to live. Thus, instead of motivating individuals to change their behavior—through education—we might argue that we could have changed the physical environment to reduce the spread of tuberculosis.

Alternatively, stepping further back in the causal chain, we might decide that the political environment in Ireland should have been the focus of intervention. If England had provided aid to the Irish during the potato blight, the Irish would not have perished in such numbers and survivors, poor and already weakened by famine, would not have been motivated to emigrate to the United States where they were highly susceptible to tuberculosis. On the other hand, going back even further, we might decide that the undiversified diet of the Irish should have been the subject of intervention. If the Irish food supply had been diversified, the potato blight would not have become a crisis for the people of that country. Again, this was a political decision on the part of the English. Thus, political strategies might be proposed that would have changed the environment, and, thus, prevented the tuberculosis epidemics of the 1850s in the United States.

The general ecological model is extremely flexible and can assume many different forms. The model becomes differentiated when a specific health problem is identified for intervention in a particular time and place. The ecological models developed beginning in the 1960s in response to the increased importance of chronic diseases made a significant departure from the classic models such as the epidemiological triangle and the wheel of causation (see Figure 1.2) used for infectious disease control and prevention. Let us explain.

Health Promotion and the Ecological Models in Public Health Since 1960

Beginning in the 1960s, the models explaining health status became increasingly limited to the behavioral determinants of health such as smoking, sedentary lifestyle, poor dietary habits, unprotected sexual activity, and failure to use seat belts, which placed the focus of public health interventions on changing individuals rather than their context. The watchwords of this trend were health promotion and disease prevention. As Green (1999) states, 1974 was a turning point when health promotion was accepted as a significant component of health policy. In a classic review of the rise in importance of health promotion, McLeroy, Bibeau, Steckler, and Glanz (1988) summarized the events and initiatives characterizing the ascendance during the 1970s and 1980s:

> Within the private sector, this interest in health promotion has led to the extensive development and implementation of health promotion programs in the worksite, increases in the marketing of 'healthy' foods, and increased societal interest in fitness. In the public sector this interest has led to national campaigns to control hypertension and cholesterol, the establishment of the Office of Disease Prevention and Health Promotion within the Public Health Service and the Center for Health Promotion and Education within the Centers for Disease Control, the development and implementation of community-wide health promotion programs by both governmental agencies and private foundations, and the establishment and monitoring of the 1990 Objectives for the Nation in health promotion. Within the professions, interest in health promotion led to the publication of the Lalonde Report in Canada, John Knowles' work on 'The Responsibility of the Individual' and the Surgeon General's report on Health Promotion/Disease Prevention in the United States, and 'Health Promotion: A Discussion Document on the Concept and Principles' in Europe. More recently, journals have appeared which are devoted exclusively to articles on health promotion programs and activities; existing journals both within and outside of traditional public health disciplines have devoted theme issues to health promotion topics; international conferences on health promotion have been held; and health education training programs have begun to focus more extensively on health promotion topics and issues. (p. 352)

The emphasis on health promotion, however, increasingly emphasized public health initiatives at the individual behavior level, rather than the environmental level. Programs to help people stop smoking, lose weight, increase exercise, eat healthier foods, and so forth proliferated, and these programs were predominantly aimed at educating and motivating individuals to change unhealthy behaviors. These initiatives were in contrast to historic interventions such as sewage disposal or food inspection that emphasized changing the environment, as we will explore in the next chapter.

PRECEDE–PROCEED and Health Promotion

By and large, health promotion programs used the now well-known model for conceptualizing community health promotion and planning: Green and Kreuter's (1991, 1999) PRECEDE–PROCEED model. The PRECEDE–PROCEED model was developed in the 1970s and has been applied, since then with a few modifications in the 1990s, which we will discuss shortly. PRECEDE stands for *P*redisposing, *R*einforcing, and *E*nabling *C*onstructs in *E*ducational *D*iagnosis and *E*valuation. Green and Kreuter (1991) define predisposing factors as:

> A person's or population's knowledge, attitudes, beliefs, values, and per-
> ceptions that facilitate or hinder motivation for change. Enabling factors
> are those skills, resources, or barriers that can help or hinder the desired
> behavioral changes as well as environmental changes. . . . Reinforcing
> factors, the rewards received, and the feedback the learner receives from
> others following adoption of the behavior, may encourage or discourage
> continuation of the behavior. (pp. 28–29)

PROCEED stands for *P*olicy, *R*egulatory, and *O*rganizational *C*onstructs in *E*ducational and *E*nvironmental *D*evelopment.

As the term *PRECEDE* denotes (predisposing, reinforcing, and enabling constructs in educational diagnosis and evaluation), the model is oriented toward improving health by changing individuals' behavior through education, and not toward intervening at the environmental level to change conditions or structures. The question structured by PRECEDE–PROCEED model is "Why do people behave badly, that is, engaging in unhealthy behaviors?" In addition, the first part of the two-art answer to this question, which is emphasized by PRECEDE–PROCEED, is lack of knowledge. Thus, education about the risks of certain behaviors and the benefits of others is a primary component of health promotion initiatives. These include initiatives to modify unfavorable dietary habits, sedentary lifestyle, substance abuse, smoking, and unsafe practices such as failure to use seat belts or follow safety precautions at work.

The second part of the answer structured by the PRECEDE–PROCEED model is related to attributes of the individual that hinder behavior change including motivation to change, appraisal of threat, self-efficacy, response efficacy, and so forth. That is, once the knowledge about health behaviors is conveyed, the challenge is to motivate individuals to change their behavior from risky to healthy. Knowledge alone is not sufficient to bring about change in health behaviors. Thus, a major tool of health promotion is the application of psychological theories to understand why people engage in unhealthy behaviors and how to stimulate them to modify these behaviors. A number of the most influential theories applied to health behavior are the Health Belief Model developed by Becker (1974); the Theory of Reasoned Action developed by Ajzen and Fishbein (1980); the Protection Motivation Theory (Rogers, 1983); Bandura's (1986) Social Cognitive Theory, which emphasizes self-efficacy; and Social Learning Theory (Rosenstock, Strecher, & Becker, 1988). These theories underlie the methods used in health promotion initiatives to motivate health behavior change.

The original PRECEDE–PROCEED model (see Figure 1.3) was described by Green in 1974 and the model he used is reproduced later in this chapter. The model visualizes the assumed causal chain, which shows that behavioral problems produce health problems, which then in turn, produce social problems, such as illegitimacy, unemployment, absenteeism, hostility, alienation, discrimination, riots, and crime. The effect of the environment on individual behavior is assumed under enabling factors such as availability of resources, accessibility, and referrals and reinforcing factors as attitudes of program personnel. However, note that this is a very restricted environment, which is limited to the immediate setting of the health education program. There is also a nonbehavioral factors box, which contributes to health problems and could contain larger environmental factors, but is not the main focus of the model and is not seen as contributing to behavior problems.

As an example of the use of the PRECEDE–PROCEED model, DeJoy (1996) describes how the model would be applied to workplace safety:

> In the PRECEDE model, three sets of diagnostic or behavioral factors drive the development of prevention strategies. Predisposing factors are the characteristics of the individual (beliefs, attitudes, values, etc.) that facilitate or hinder self-protective behavior. Predisposing factors are conceptualized as providing the motivation for behavior. The threat-related beliefs and efficacy expectancies that are prominent features of the value-expectancy models (psychological theories for health behavior) would be included here. Enabling factors refer to objective aspects of the

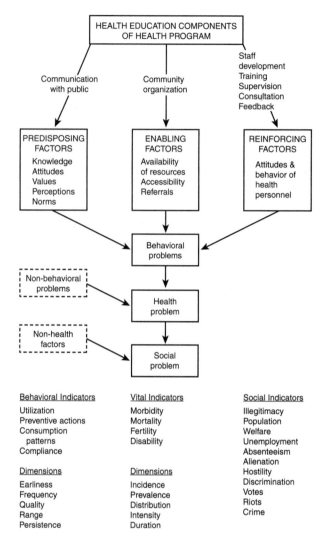

FIGURE 1.3   Approximate relationships among "objects of interest" in the planning and evaluation of health education from *Health Education Monographs*.

environment or system that block or promote self-protective action. Green and colleagues define enabling factors as "factors antecedent to behavior that allow motivation or aspiration to be realized." The skill and knowledge necessary to follow prescribed actions would be included here, as would the availability and accessibility of protective equipment and other resources. Most barriers or costs would be classified as enabling factors. Reinforcing factors involve any reward or punishment that follows or is anticipated as a consequence of the behavior. Performance feedback and the social approval/disapproval received from coworkers, supervisors, and managers would qualify as reinforcing factors in workplace settings. (p. 66)

Clearly, the target for intervention in this example is the worker and his or her motivation to avoid workplace injuries. This orientation is apparent, when the author describes the predisposing factors as "providing the motivation for behavior," and also includes worker's psychological factors such as beliefs about threat and efficacy. Enabling factors "allow motivation or aspiration to be realized" include the worker's skill and knowledge. It is plain that the intervention strategy is to induce the practice of safety through education that enables the worker; application of psychological theories that address the worker's predisposing attitudes, beliefs, and values related to safety practices; and rewards or punishments that reinforce the worker's safety-related behavior.

Importantly, the environment—in this case, the physical workplace and the people who manage it—is seen as reinforcing and enabling the worker to engage in safety habits, but not as the target of the intervention. Rather, improving workplace safety is focused on motivating the individual worker to practice safety habits, not motivating the employer or the larger society to modify the workplace. The individual worker's motivation to practice workplace safety is the subject of the intervention, and the worker is viewed as the accountable party.

Also, note that the environment is quite proscribed. Its bounds are the specific workplace itself. The environment, in this example, does not include larger political and economic factors that may affect what occurs within the workplace. For instance, the political and economic factors that impact the availability of protective equipment and other resources required for safety are not considered. Regulations governing safety in the workplace are not considered, nor are the enforcement of regulations. This example is typical of health promotion programs, particularly through the 1990s. The larger environment could certainly be incorporated into the model, but it usually was not.

Why Health Promotion?

The health promotion trend, whereby the target of public health interventions was individuals' behavior instead of the environment, was, in part, because of the view that the distal causes of poor health—physical and social environmental factors including cultural, economic, and political—were too difficult to change.

Also, health promotion was tied to the desire for health care cost containment. Educating individuals about health was seen as a way to make people more self-sufficient in health, engage in self-care, and become better informed consumers of health services. Because of concern about spiraling health care costs in the 1960s and onward, health promotion was presented as a means to control costs through the demand side (Green, 1999). This can be seen in the proliferation of research studies undertaken to improve health care utilization and decrease unhealthy behaviors through educational interventions for patients/consumers:

It caused them to reason by analogy from medical successes that our scientific quest should be to find the best intervention to achieve a specific type of health-related behavior change. Practitioners and the agencies funding health services and public health research eagerly embraced this search for magic-bullet solutions to the behavioral change problems presented by medical care and public health. A generation of highly controlled randomized trials and fine-grained behavioral research ensued. These tested, by trial and error, specific ways to improve patient compliance. They included ways to reduce broken appointments, educate mothers to restrain their tendency to bring a child to health maintenance organization or pediatric services for each earache or sore throat, improve smoking cessation, and modify a range of specific consumer and self-care behaviors. The targets of the magic bullet interventions were as much those behaviors thought to account for some of the unnecessary and inappropriate uses of health services as those accounting for leading causes of death or disability. (p. 75)

It was also apparent that individual behaviors such as smoking, sedentary lifestyle, and poor dietary habits were highly related to the onset and progression of chronic diseases such as heart disease, pulmonary disease, and diabetes. If risky health behaviors could be changed, it was argued, the incidence of chronic diseases would be reduced. Of course, this is true.

The question, however, is whether trying to motivate individuals to change their behavior—through education, incentives, and disincentives—is the most effective and just means of accomplishing this goal. Is placing accountability for behavior change onto the individual, without changing the environment in which that behavior occurs, realistic and fair?

Criticisms of Health Promotion

Placing the locus of accountability for poor health on the individual is one of the major criticisms of the health promotion movement. Viewing the individual's behavior as the problem to be "fixed," rather than the context in which that behavior occurs, is seen as "blaming the victim." Under this view, the context of people's lives structure their health behaviors to a large degree, and so blaming individuals for having poor health behaviors is ineffective and unfair. For example, poor people and those of minority groups often live in neighborhoods with supermarkets that carry limited amounts of healthy foods, especially fruits and vegetables. Their shelves predominate, instead, with high-fat, high-sodium snack foods that have little nutritional value (Moore & Roux, 2006). Does the fairer and more effective public health intervention, aimed at improving the diet of people in such neighborhoods, target the residents themselves or the supermarkets? These are the kinds of questions that arise from the debate over the PRECEDE–PROCEED model.

Not surprisingly, beginning in the 1980s, the pendulum began to swing back to a focus on environmentally targeted interventions and an interest in understanding the interaction between individuals and their environment. Because of the "blaming-the-victim" argument, as well as the recognition that health education was not as effective as it had once been thought to be, interest in alternatives to the health promotion approach intensified. As Green himself noted in 1999, "The dominant emphasis has shifted from psychological and behavioral factors, which lend themselves to precise measure, to more difficult to measure and control factors, such as social, cultural, and political ones" (Green & Kreuter, 1999, p. 8). Further:

> In 1986, the First International Conference on Health Promotion produced the Ottawa Charter, which helped reorient policy, programs, and practices away from these proximal risk factors. The shift that followed was to the more distal risk factors in time, space, or scope, which we shall call risk conditions. These also influence health, either through the risk factors or by operating directly on human biology over time, but they are less likely than risk factors to be under the control of the individual at risk. (p. 10)

Consistent with the pendulum swing, Green and Kreuter revised the PRECEDE–PROCEED model (see Figure 1.4) in 1991 to place more emphasis on the context of behavior. With respect to incorporating

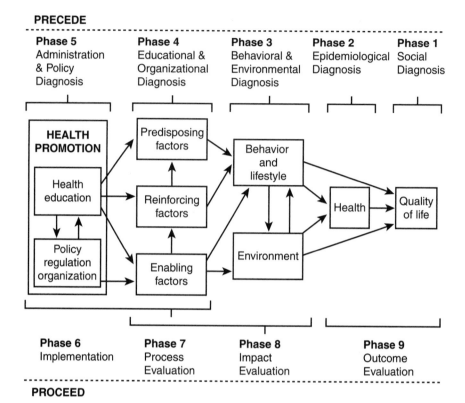

PRECEDE

Phase 5	Phase 4	Phase 3	Phase 2	Phase 1
Administration & Policy Diagnosis	Educational & Organizational Diagnosis	Behavioral & Environmental Diagnosis	Epidemiological Diagnosis	Social Diagnosis

Phase 6	Phase 7	Phase 8	Phase 9
Implementation	Process Evaluation	Impact Evaluation	Outcome Evaluation

PROCEED

FIGURE 1.4   The PRECEDE-PROCEED model for health promotion planning and evaluation. From Green & Kreuter, 1999, *Health Promotion Planning, 3rd edition.*

environmental influences, the model now contains a box labeled *environment*, which notably both influences and is influenced by behavior and lifestyle. This change in the PRECEDE–PROCEED model now makes it in keeping with the general ecological model, which assumes that individuals are affected by their environment. In addition, the model now includes a policy regulation organization factor, which impacts the enabling factors and, through these, the environment. The main features and causal assumptions of the 1974 PRECEDE–PROCEED model remain the same— predisposing, reinforcing, and enabling factors affect behavior and lifestyle, which in turn, impact health.

In 1999, Green and Kreuter made minor modifications to the PRECEDE–PROCEED model, and enlarged the role of the environment in their description of the factors influencing behavior. The risk factors and risk conditions, together with factors predisposing, enabling, and reinforcing them, are referred to in the PRECEDE–PROCEED model collectively as the determinants of health.

> These include adequate housing; secure income; healthful and safe community and work environment; enforcement of policies and regulations controlling the manufacture, marketing, labeling, and sale of potentially harmful products; and the use of these products (such as alcohol and tobacco) where they can harm others. (p. 10)

Although the revised model placed more emphasis on the environment, the focus was still on providing a blueprint for changing the individual's behavior through education and relying on psychological theories for understanding how to motivate behavioral change. The context was identified in the model as necessary to achieve individual behavioral changes. However, in practice, changes to the context within health promotion programs were usually still limited and proscribed to the immediate setting. They did not aim to change underlying social structures or other larger environmental factors.

Population Health and Reemphasis of the Social Environment in Public Health Models

At the same time that health promotion was coming under attack, the population health approach was introduced and began to gain followers in the field of public health. Stirred by antipathy toward the emphasis on interventions that used education and psychologically based strategies to motivate individuals to change their behavior rather than changing the context or structure in which behavior occurs, this approach to public health focused on the distal social environment—power, wealth, and status—as the root cause of health problems. The evidence supporting this approach is the large body of research on disparities or inequalities in health status between the rich and the poor, the powerful and powerless, and those of high social status and those of low status. Incontrovertible findings that an individual's social status, wealth, and power have a profound influence on his or her chances of being healthy underwrite the population health approach to public health. The Whitehall study was one of the first to demonstrate what has become a consistent finding— people who are structurally disadvantaged are far more likely than the advantaged to have poor health.

Studies have asked, "Why do some people exercise and others do not?" "Why do some people eat nutritious foods and others do not?" "Why do some people lead sedentary lives and others do not?" "Why do some communities have support groups for behavior change and others do not?" "Why do some communities have opportunities for exercise and relaxation and others do not?" "Why are some communities free from toxic substances in the environment and others are not?" The answer is in the unequal distribution of power, wealth, and status that give the advantaged the opportunities and resources to live in healthier environments, engage in healthier behaviors, and have access to better health care.

As Marmot (2005) states,

> The gross inequalities in health that we see within and between countries present a challenge to the world. That there should be a spread of life expectancy of 48 years among countries and 20 years or more within countries is not inevitable. A burgeoning volume of research identifies social factors (i.e., wealth, power, and status) at the root of much of these inequalities in health. Social determinants are relevant to communicable and non-communicable disease alike. (p. 1099)

The population health approach has led to studies such as the following by Pickard, Miller, and Kirkpatrick (2009) that offer explanations for undesirable health behaviors in terms of the social context of the individual. That is, the social context is viewed as having a causal impact on health behaviors.

Social determinants of health are widely described but few researchers have more than cursory contact with those whose lives fall into the most impoverished, epidemiological categories. Framing the problems as inappropriate emergency room visits and non-compliance with treatment regimens sheds little light on the choices driving such behaviors. Drawing on 11 years of working continually among residents of a highly diverse and grindingly poor urban neighborhood, this paper examines the meanings people assign to their health behaviors. It presents a new "care seeking typology" based on a content analysis of accounts shared in nearly 400 in-depth neighborhood interviews. When combined with close observations of patients in a small university affiliated, community based safety-net clinic, 10 health seeker types emerge. Each type is illustrated with authentic stories rarely surfaced by traditional scientific methods and validated through reviews by community participants. While several resulting composites mirror frequently cited stereotypes of downtrodden lives, others challenge prevailing beliefs about why and how the poor make health care decisions. Not surprisingly, money plays a central role in care seeking among the population studied. However, the connection is frequently misunderstood by health providers and policymakers, with frustratingly predictable results. Opportunities for more successful therapeutic engagement emerge from this new mapping of social perceptions. (Pickard, Miller, & Kirkpatrick, 2009)

The population health perspective is leading to more complex public health models that integrate distal and proximal social factors, physical environmental factors, and behavioral factors to predict disease, disability, and premature death. Health behaviors are viewed as patterned by the social environment, not "free-standing" (Chan, Gordon, Chong, & Alter, 2008; Purslow et al., 2008). For example, a recent study of the original Whitehall participants who have been followed for 24 years (Stringhini et al., 2010) investigated the role of health behaviors in the relationship between socioeconomic position and mortality. The behaviors studied included smoking, alcohol consumption, diet, and physical activity. The authors found that "there was an association between socioeconomic position and mortality that was substantially accounted for by adjustment for health behaviors, particularly when the behaviors were assess repeatedly." (p. 1159)

Among champions of population health, the commitment to social justice is at the heart of public health's promise.

Health disparities/inequalities include differences between the most advantaged group in a given category – e.g., the wealthiest, the most powerful racial/ethnic group – and all others, not only between the best- and worst-off groups. Pursuing health equity means pursuing the elimination of such health disparities/inequalities. (Braveman, 2006, p. 167)

Everyone, not only the rich, the powerful, or those with social standing, is entitled to the conditions that produce health. It is in the tradition of public health to advocate for those who have unequal access to opportunities and resources in society as well as those with advantages, following in the footsteps of the public health engineering era when people in all stations of life were provided with clean water, sewage and garbage disposal, and a clean food supply in the cities of industrializing nations.

Summary

Over the last 50 years, the emphasis of public health initiatives on behavior, rather than on environment, became widespread. Even though the ecological approach of public health views the individual as embedded in a physical and social environment and affected by it, the health promotion orientation led to an emphasis on behavior and a de-emphasis on the environment—both physical and social. The recent President's Cancer Panel (2010) report provides an example of the divergence in orientation that has occurred and still exists. The report, *Reducing Environmental Cancer Risk: What We Can Do Now*, is unlike previous president's reports, which focused on individual behaviors, diagnosis, and treatment rather than the risk of environmental exposures. The 2010 report found that "A growing body of research documents myriad established and suspected environmental factors linked to genetic, immune, and endocrine dysfunction that can lead to cancer and other diseases." The panel advised that the "true burden of environmentally induced cancers has been grossly underestimated, " and that the current estimates of 2% of all cancers caused by environmental toxins and 4% by occupational exposures is outdated. Of the more than 80,000 chemical used in the United States today, only a few hundred have been tested for health effects. Environmental contaminants come from industrial and manufacturing processes, agriculture, household products, medical technologies, military practices, and the natural environment. The report argues that the problem has not been addressed adequately by the National Cancer Program, which has focused on individual behaviors, screening, diagnosis, and treatment. It finds the current regulatory approach reactionary rather than precautionary—a substance's danger must be demonstrated incontrovertibly before action is taken to reduce exposure to it. Therefore, the "public bears the burden of proving that a given environmental exposure is harmful" (President's Cancer Panel, p. ii).

The still-existing tension between those who emphasize behavioral and those who emphasize environmental causes is demonstrated in the reaction to the 2010 President's Report. The panel urged the president to act on its findings, but the reaction to the report was critical from Michael Thun, vice president of Epidemiology and Surveillance Research at the American Cancer Society, who tried to bring the focus back to behavior. As reported in *The New York Times* (Grady, 2010), Dr. Thun stated that the report was

"unbalanced by its implication that pollution is the major cause of cancer." . . . Suggesting that the risk is much higher, when there is no proof, may divert attention from things that are much bigger causes of cancer, like smoking. "If we could get rid of tobacco, we could get rid of 30 percent of cancer deaths," he said, adding that poor nutrition, obesity, and lack of exercise are also greater contributors to cancer risk than pollution.

This discussion exemplifies some of the complexities of taking a primary prevention approach to health, that is, to prevent health problems from beginning. There are many choices made when determining how to improve or maintain health, and one is the choice of an individual- or environmental-level intervention. Given the premise of the ecological model—that individuals are embedded in an environment, which they both influence and are influenced by—both components of the model are relevant. Within the ecological model, both the individual and the context are potential sites of public health interventions, and both have been employed throughout the history of public health. For example, in the early part of the 20th century, there were interventions that focused on the individual level—teaching and encouraging individuals in immigrant communities to engage in certain health behaviors such as hand washing that prevent infectious diseases—and those that focused on the environmental level, notably the environmental engineering interventions that brought clean water, safe food supply, and sanitary disposal of waste to these communities and also prevented the spread of infectious diseases. The emphasis on environmental over individual-level interventions changes over time, as we have seen in the discussion of public health models since 1960. Neither approach is ever entirely abandoned, but in different eras, one may be emphasized over the other. Indeed, a study of tuberculosis control in the 19th and 20th centuries led Fairchild and Oppenheimer (1998) to argue for a more nuanced approach to public health practice in which strategies that address both individual and environmental causes of disease with broad and targeted interventions are employed: "If the relative contribution of different interventions and factors is to be sorted out, pursuit of mono-causal explanations for the retreat of TB, like monotypic intervention, is insufficient" (p. 1113).

These and other decisions about how to promote and maintain health in populations go to the heart of public health practice. Public health, as a field, plans and initiates prevention activities— primary, secondary, and tertiary. However, many important choices about these activities translate the public health mission into public health practice. Several choices are central to the actuality of public health:

- What health problems are addressed?
- Where are interventions targeted—environmental, individual, or multilevel?
- If targeted at the environmental level, are interventions focused on distal or proximal factors?
- Are methods voluntary or coercive?
- Are activities public or private enterprises?
- If private, are activities nonprofit or profit making?

To clarify these choices and how they impact practice, we can examine the provision of clean water in the United States. Although water treatment has been practiced throughout human history as far back as 2000 BC in ancient Greece and India, before the mid-1850s, the motivation to treat water, usually with some form of filtering, was to improve taste and reduce turbidity. In the mid-1800s, the need to treat water to prevent infectious disease outbreaks was beginning to be understood, even before we knew that water could contain microorganisms that caused these diseases. How water became associated with specific diseases is the story of one of the most famous public health achievements—John Snow's identification, through application of epidemiological principles, of the Broad Street pump as the source of the 1853 cholera epidemic in London. Here is the story as told by Judith Summers (1989):

When a wave of Asiatic cholera first hit England in late 1831, it was thought to be spread by "miasma in the atmosphere." By the time of the Soho outbreak 23 years later, medical knowledge about the disease had barely changed, though one man, Dr John Snow, a surgeon [actually an anesthesiologist] and pioneer of the science of epidemiology, had recently published a report speculating that it was spread by contaminated water—an idea with which neither the authorities nor the rest of the medical profession had much truck. Whenever cholera broke out—which it did four times between 1831 and 1854—nothing whatsoever was done to contain it, and it rampaged through the industrial cities, leaving tens of thousands dead in its wake. The year 1853 saw outbreaks in Newcastle and Gateshead as well as in London, where a total of 10,675 people died of the disease. In the 1854 London epidemic the worst-hit areas at first were Southwark and Lambeth. Soho suffered only a few, seemingly isolated, cases in late August. Then, on the night of the 31st, what Dr Snow later called "the most terrible outbreak of cholera which ever occurred in the kingdom" broke out.

It was as violent as it was sudden. During the next three days, 127 people living in or around Broad Street died. Few families, rich or poor, were spared the loss of at least one member. Within a week, three-quarters of the residents had fled from their homes, leaving their shops shuttered, their houses locked and the streets deserted. Only those who could not afford to leave remained there. It was like the Great Plague all over again.

By 10 September, the number of fatal attacks had reached 500 and the death rate of the St Anne's, Berwick Street and Golden Square subdivisions of the parish had risen to 12.8 per cent—more than double that for the rest of London. That it did not rise even higher was thanks only to Dr John Snow.

Snow lived in Frith Street, so his local contacts made him ideally placed to monitor the epidemic which had broken out on his doorstep. His previous researches had convinced him that cholera, which, as he had noted, "always commences with disturbances of the functions of the alimentary canal," was spread by a poison passed from victim to victim through sewage-tainted water; and he had traced a recent outbreak in South London to contaminated water supplied by the Vauxhall Water Company—a theory that the authorities and the water company itself were, not surprisingly, reluctant to believe. Now he saw his chance to prove his theories once and for all, by linking the Soho outbreak to a single source of polluted water.

From day one he patrolled the district, interviewing the families of the victims. His research led him to a pump on the corner of Broad Street and Cambridge Street, at the epicenter of the epidemic. "I found," he wrote afterwards, "that nearly all the deaths had taken place within a short distance of the pump." In fact, in houses much nearer another pump, there had only been 10 deaths — and of those, five victims had always drunk the water from the Broad Street pump, and three were schoolchildren, who had probably drunk from the pump on their way to school.

Dr. Snow took a sample of water from the pump, and, on examining it under a microscope, found that it contained "white, flocculent particles." By 7 September, he was convinced that these were the source of infection, and he took his findings to the Board of Guardians of St James's Parish, in whose parish the pump fell.

Though they were reluctant to believe him, they agreed to remove the pump handle as an experiment. When they did so, the spread of cholera dramatically stopped. [Actually the outbreak had already lessened for several days.]. (pp. 113–117)

Knowledge about disease-causing microorganisms increased dramatically during the remainder of the 19th century because of advances in the microscope and other instruments. Cholera, typhoid, hepatitis, and other infectious diseases were understood to be waterborne and controllable through water treatment. Because of the tremendous death toll from such diseases, by the advent of the 20th century, water purification was considered an important public health issue, and methods to provide clean water were underway. The filtration systems of the past had been somewhat, but not entirely, effective against waterborne diseases. The first widely used method to eliminate waterborne disease organisms was chlorination. In 1970, public health concerns shifted from waterborne illnesses caused by microorganisms, to water pollution from pesticide residues, industrial waste, and organic chemicals. Regulations and water treatment plants were developed to respond to this source of water contamination as well (Jesperson, 2004).

In the United States as in many other countries, providing clean water was viewed as a public good or utility. As a result, government at every level invested in water purification systems, and water treatment became a staple public health service. Government regulations set standards for water used for human consumption, and clean water was provided throughout the country by public or publicly regulated organizations. The exceptions were for people who lived in remote areas and obtained their water from private wells.

With respect to public health choices about how to improve health, this approach to preventing waterborne infectious diseases may be viewed as an archetypical primary prevention; purifying water supplies is intended to prevent infectious diseases such as cholera, typhoid, and hepatitis from occurring at all. As for the strategy chosen to prevent waterborne infectious diseases, water treatment systems such as those in the United States are environmental-level interventions. Our systems of preventing exposure to unclean water do not depend on individual behaviors such as boiling water or adding chlorine to water for individual use. Under the environmental-level approach that we have followed, clean water is delivered to individuals through a system that is planned, installed, monitored, and maintained by an organization, irrespective of an individual user's actions. Using and/or creating clean water is not the responsibility of the individual. In addition, the water treatment organization in the United States is generally a public utility, not a private enterprise.

HEALTH IMPACT PYRAMID

The health impact pyramid developed by Frieden (2010) provides a very useful framework for integrating these ideas into public health practice (See Figure 1. 5). "A 5-tier pyramid best describes the impact of different types of public health interventions and provides a framework to improve health. At the base of this pyramid, indicating interventions with the greatest potential impact, are efforts to address socio-economic determinants of health. In ascending order are interventions that change the context to make individuals' default decisions healthy, clinical interventions that require limited contact but confer long-term protection, and ongoing directly clinical care, and health education and counseling" (Frieden, 2010, p. 590). Note that the author accepts the population

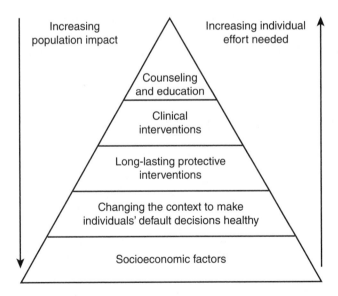

FIGURE 1.5   The Health Impact Pyramid. From Frieden, T. R. (2010). A framework for public health action: The health impact pyramid. *American Journal of Public Health*, 100, 591.

health perspective that structural inequality embodied in socioeconomic factors is the level with the most potential to improve health—a primary prevention strategy. Also note that the second level—changing the context—is a primary prevention strategy, which includes provision of clean water and safe food, as well as passage of laws that prevent injuries and exposure to disease-producing agents. Interventions at the top tiers are a mix of primary, secondary, and tertiary prevention "designed to help individuals, rather than entire populations, but they could theoretically have a large population impact if universally and effectively applied. In practice, however, even the best programs at the pyramid's higher levels achieve limited public health impact, largely because of their dependence on long-term individual behavior change" (Frieden, 2010, p. 591).

In the following chapters, we will discuss the practice of public health. We will examine what public health practitioners actually do and how their practice relates to the mission of public health and to primary, secondary, and tertiary prevention. So far, we have discussed public health in the ideal. However, the actual practice of public health does not always attain the ideal. In the next set of chapters, we will discuss the public health system as it is currently practiced in the United States and its historical origins. This will involve discussing the components of the public health system, including organization, financing, management, and performance, as well as the health problems that are addressed by public health. In this review, we will see how public health practice today in the United States compares to the ideal of "assuring conditions in which people can be healthy."

THE PROSPECTS FOR PUBLIC HEALTH

In the final chapter of the book, we will discuss the prospects for the field of public health.

The promise of public health rests on social justice—everyone is entitled to the conditions that can maintain health. In practice, public health is a loose confederation of organizations and public agencies that are often not in a position to maintain or create the conditions that lead to health. Therefore, what are the prospects for public health? What conditions can public health affect? There is evidence that public health practice is on the cusp of change that will return the field to more politically oriented action aimed at changing underlying structures of society that maintain inequalities throughout the world in morbidity, disability, and premature death between rich and poor, powerful and powerless, and high and low status. As Marmot (2005) writes:

> Health status, therefore, should be of concern to policy makers in every sector, not solely those involved in health policy. As a response to this global challenge, WHO (World Health Organization) is launching a Commission on Social Determinants of Health, which will review the evidence, raise societal debate, and recommend policies with the goal of improving health of the world's most vulnerable people. A major thrust of the commission is turning public health knowledge into political action. (p. 1099)

On the other hand, the pressure to continue emphasizing interventions that motivate people to change their behavior through traditional health promotion has wide support because it does not challenge existing power structures. It will be easier to maintain a focus on motivating individuals to change their own behavior, rather than taking on the difficult task of providing, in the broadest sense, the conditions in which people can be healthy. These issues will be considered in the final chapter.

Another issue will be who will provide public health services. Much of the work of public health is done by the public sector, but as the Institute of Medicine emphasized in The Future of the Public's Health in the 21st Century, public health extends beyond government to encompass, "the efforts, science, art, and approaches used by all sectors of society (public, private, and civil society) to assure, maintain, protect, promote, and improve the health of the people" (IOM, 2003). Consistent with this view, public health "can be seen as an ideology, a profession, a movement, or a set of actions, but not as a single scientific discipline" (Savitz, Poole, & Miller, 1999).

For example, we, in the United States, where access to clean water is guaranteed by public utilities through environmental-level structures that deliver potable water to individuals in their homes, worksites, and public places, may assume that our system was the only way the goal of providing water free from disease-producing agents could have been achieved. However, this is not the case. Other models have been developed and are being tried throughout the world, mostly in poor countries and poor communities. They include water systems developed by the private sector such as in Bolivia, where the government licensed water distribution in the 1990s to private companies, headed by Bechtel (Salzman, 2006). Alternate strategies include individual-level strategies whereby people are responsible for filtering their own water using small-scale technologies such as the UV Waterworks, a portable, low-maintenance, energy-efficient water purifier, uses ultraviolet light to render viruses and bacteria harmless (National Academy of Engineering, 2010). They include the Acumen Fund water initiatives that provide potable water in poor countries using market-based concepts and private investment without government help (Acumen Fund, 2010). These alternative strategies to providing potable water that is free from water-borne disease agents illustrate the variety of ways that public health problems can be addressed.

However, the questions that must be raised about the selection of strategies to achieve public health goals are related to their effectiveness, efficiency, and equity.

The purpose of this book is to open the field of public health to those new to it. Many complexities are not discussed in this attempt to make the overall values, goals, and practices of the field accessible to those unfamiliar with public health. With broad strokes, we hope to develop in the reader an appreciation of public health and an interest in learning more about the challenges and complexities of providing conditions in which people can be healthy.

REFERENCES

Acumen Fund. (2010). *Water portfolio*. Retrieved July 7, 2010, from http://www .acumenfund.org/investments/portfolios/water-portfolio.html

Ajzen, I., & Fishbein, M. (1980). *Understanding attitudes and predicting social behavior*. Englewood Cliffs, NJ: Prentice-Hall.

Bandura, A. (1986). *Social foundations of thought and action: A social cognitive theory*. Englewood Cliff, NJ: Prentice-Hall.

Becker, M. H. (1974). *The health belief model and personal health behavior*. Thorofare, NJ: C. B. Slack.

Berkman L. F., & Glass T. (2000). Social integration, social networks, social support, and health. In L. F. Berkman & I. Kawachi (Eds.), *Social epidemiology* (pp. 137–173). Oxford, UK: Oxford University Press.

Braveman, P. (2006). Health disparities and health equity: Concepts and measurement. *Annual Review of Public Health, 27*, 167–194.

Centers for Disease Control and Prevention. (2003). *Environmental public health indicators*. Atlanta, GA: National Center for Environmental Health, Division of Environmental Hazards and Health Effects.

Centers for Disease Control and Prevention. (2010a). *Multistate outbreak of E. coli O157:H7 infections associated with beef from National Steak and Poultry*. Retrieved April 19, 2010, from http://www.cdc.gov/ecoli/2010/index.html

Centers for Disease Control and Prevention.(2010b). *Deaths, percent of total deaths, and death rates for the 15 leading causes of death: United States and each state, 1999–2006*. Retrieved May 2, 2010, from http://www.cdc.gov/nchs/nvss/mortality/lcwk9.htm

Chan, R. H., Gordon, N. F., Chong, A., Alter, D. A., & Socioeconomic and Acute Myocardial Infarction Investigators. (2008). Influence of socioeconomic status on lifestyle behavior modifications among survivors of acute myocardial infarction. *American Journal of Cardiology, 102*(12), 1583–1588.

Cohen, S. (2004). Social relationships and health. *American Psychologist, 59*, 676–684.

DeJoy, D. (1996). Theoretical models of health behavior and workplace self-protective behavior. *Journal of Safety Research, 27*(2), 61–72.

Dooley, D., Fielding J., & Levi L. (1996). Health and unemployment. *Annual Review of Public Health, 17*, 449–465.

Dubos, R. (1959). *Mirage of health: Utopias, progress, and biological change*. New York: Harper & Brothers.

Evans, R. G., & Stoddart, G. L. (1994). Producing health, consuming health care. In R. G. Evans, M. L. Barer, & T. R. Marmor (Eds.), *Why are some people healthy and others not?* New York: Aldine de Gruyter.

Fairchild, A. L., & Oppenheimer, G. M. (1998). Public health nihilism vs pragmatism: History, politics, and the control of tuberculosis. *American Journal of Public Health, 88*(7), 1105–1117.

Fos, P. J., & Fine, D. J. (2000). *Designing health care for populations: Applied epidemiology in health care administration*. San Francisco: Jossey-Bass.

Frieden, T. R. (2010). A framework for public health action: The health impact pyramid. *American Journal of Public Health, 100*, 590–595.

Friis, R. H., & Sellers, T. A. (1996). *Epidemiology for public health practice*. Gaithersburg, MD: Aspen.

Grady, D. (May 6, 2010). U.S. panel criticized as overstating cancer risks. *The New York Times*.

Green, L. W. (1974). Toward cost-benefit evaluations of health education: Some concepts, methods, and examples. *Health Education Monographs, 2*(Supp. 1), 34–64.

Green, L. W. (1999). Health education's contributions to public health in the twentieth century: A glimpse through health promotion's rear-view mirror. *Annual Review of Public Health, 20*, 67–88.

Green, L. W., & Kreuter, M. W. (1991). *Health promotion planning* (2nd ed.). Palo Alto, CA: Mayfield Publishing.

Green, L. W., & Kreuter, M. W. (1999). *Health promotion planning: An educational and ecological approach* (3rd ed.). Palo Alto, CA: Mayfield Publishing.

Institute of Medicine (IOM). (1988). The future of public health. Washington, DC: *National Academy Press*.

Jesperson, K. (2010). *Search for clean water continues.* Retrieved July 7, 2010, from http://www.nesc.wvu.edu/old_website/ndwc/ndwc_DWH_1.html

Kaplan, B. H., Cassel, J. C., & Gore, S. (1977). Social support and health. *Medical Care, 15*(5 Suppl.), 47–58.

Karasek, R., Baker, D., Marxer, F., Ahlbom, A., & Theorell, T. (1981). Job decision latitude, job demands, and cardiovascular disease: A prospective study of Swedish men. *American Journal of Public Health, 71*(7), 694–705.

Karasek, R., Brisson, C., Kawakami, N., Houtman, I., Bongers, P., & Amick, B. (1998). The Job Content Questionnaire: An instrument for internationally comparative assessments of psychosocial job characteristics. *Journal of Occupational Health Psychology, 3*(4), 322–355.

Kasl, S. V., & Jones, B. A. (2000). The impact of job loss and retirement on health. In L. F. Berkman & I. Kawachi (Eds.), *Social epidemiology* (pp. 118–136). Oxford, UK: Oxford University Press.

Kasl, S. V., Rodriguez, E., & Lasch K. E. (1998). The impact of unemployment on health and well-being. In B. P. Dohrenwend (Ed.), *Adversity, stress, and psychopathology* (pp. 111–131). New York: Oxford University Press.

Krieger, N. (2000). Discrimination and health. In: L. F. Berkman & I. Kawachi (Eds.). *Social epidemiology* (36–75). Oxford, UK: Oxford University Press.

Krieger, N., & Birn, A. E. (1998). A vision of social justice as the foundation of public health: Commemorating 150 years of the spirit of 1848. *American Journal of Public Health, 88*(11), 1603–1606.

Lasagna, L. (1970). *The doctors' dilemmas.* New York: Harper & Row. As reported on the University of California San Francisco School of Medicine, Agents of Change http://medschool2.ucsf.edu/spotlights/agents-change.

Lynch, J. W., Smith, G. D., Kaplan, G. A., & House, J. S. (2000). Income inequality and mortality: Importance to health of individual income, psychosocial environment, or material conditions. *British Medical Journal, 320*, 1200–1204.

Mays, V. M., Cochran, S. D., and Barnes, N. W. (2007). Race, race-based discrimination, and health outcomes among african americans, *Annual Review of Psychology, 58*, 201–225.

Marmot, M. (2005). Social determinants of health inequalities. *Lancet, 365*(9464), 1099–1104.

Marmot, M. G., Bobak, M., & Smith, G. D. (1995). Explanations for social inequalities in health. In B. C. Amick III, S. Levine, A. R. Tarlov, & D. C. Walsh (Eds.), *Society and health.* New York: Oxford University Press.

McGinnis, J. M., & Foege W. H. (1993). Actual causes of death in the United States. *Journal of the American Medical Association, 270,* 2207–2212.

McGinnis, J. M., Williams-Russo, P., & Knickman, J. R. (2002). The case for more active policy attention to health promotion. *Health Affairs, 21,* 78–93.

McLeroy, K. R., Bibeau, D., Steckler, A, & Glanz, K. (1988). An ecological perspective on health promotion programs. *Health Education Quarterly, 15*(4), 351–377.

Moore, L. V., & Roux, A. V. D. (2006). Associations of neighborhood characteristics with the location and type of food stores. *American Journal of Public Health, 96*(2), 325–331.

National Academy of Engineering. (2010). Water supply and distribution timeline. Retrieved July 8, 2010, from http://www.greatachievements.org/?id=3610

Pencheon D., Guest C., Melzer D., & Gray, J. A. M. (Eds.). (2001). *Oxford handbook of public health practice.* Oxford, New York: Oxford University Press.

Peterson, R. K. D. (1995). Insects, disease, and military history: The Napoleonic campaigns and historical perception. *American Entomologist, 41,* 147–160.

Pickard, R. B., Miller, A. N., & Kirkpatrick, F. (2009). A decade on the mean streets: A new typology for understanding health choices of those living in poverty's grasp. Philadelphia, PA: American Public Health Association Annual Meeting.

President's Cancer Panel, National Cancer Institute. (April, 2010). *Reducing environmental cancer risk: What we can do now.* Washington, DC: U.S. Department of Health and Human Services, National Institutes of Health.

Prochaska, J. O., & DiClemente C. C. (1982). Transtheoretical therapy: Toward a more integrative model of change. *Psychotherapy: Theory, research, and practice, 20,* 161–173.

Purslow L. R., Young E. H., Wareham N. J., Forouhi N., Brunner E. J., Luben R. N., et al. (2008). Socioeconomic position and risk of short-term weight gain: Prospective study of 14,619 middle-aged men and women. *BMC Public Health, 8,* 112.

Rogers, R. W. (1983). Cognitive and psychological processes in fear appeals and attitude change: A revised theory of protection motivation. In J. T. Cacioppo & R. E. Petty (Eds.), *Social psychophysiology: A sourcebook* (pp. 153–176). New York: Guilford Press.

Rosenstock, I. M, Strecher, V. J. & Becker, M. H (1988). Social learning theory and the health belief model. *Health Education Quarterly, 15*(2), 175–183.

Salzman, J. (2006). Thirst: A short history of drinking water. *Duke Law Faculty Scholarship.* Paper 1261. Retrieved July 7, 2010, from http://scholarship.law.duke.edu/faculty_scholarship/1261

Samet, J. M., Marbury, M. C., & Spengler, J. D. (1987). Health effects and sources of indoor air pollution. Part 1. *American Review of Respiratory Diseases, 136,* 1486–1508.

Smedley, B. D., Stith, A. Y. & Nelson, A. R. (Eds.). (2003). *Unequal treatment: Confronting racial and ethnic disparities in health care.* Washington, DC: National Academies Press.

Stokols, D. (1996). Translating social ecological theory into guidelines for community health promotion. *American Journal of Health Promotion, 10*(4), 282–298.

Stringhini, S., Sabia, S., Shipley, M., Brunner, E., Nabi, H., Kivimaki, M., et al. (2010). Association of socioeconomic position with health behaviors and mortality. *Journal of the American Medical Association, 303*(12), 1159–1166.

Summers, J. (1989). *Soho—A history of London's most colourful neighborhood.* London: Bloomsbury Pub.

Theorell, T. (2000). Working conditions and health. In L. F. Berkman & I. Kawachi (Eds.), *Social epidemiology* (pp. 95–117). Oxford, UK: Oxford University Press.

Thoits, P. A. (1982). Life stress, social support, and psychological vulnerability: Epidemiological considerations. *Journal of Community Psychology, 10*(4), 341–362.

U.S. Department of Health and Human Services. (1998). Call to action: Eliminating racial and ethnic disparities in health. Potomac, MD: Author.

U.S. Department of Health and Human Services. (2010). *Find shortage areas: MUA/P by state and county.* Retrieved April 19, 2010, from http://muafind .hrsa.gov/

World Health Organization. (1946). *Preamble to the Constitution of the World Health Organization* as adopted by the International Health Conference, New York, June 19–22, 1946; signed on July 22, 1946, by the representatives of 61 states (Official Records of the World Health Organization, no. 2, p. 100) and entered into force on April 7, 1948.

World Health Organization. (2010). *The determinants of health.* Retrieved April 23, 2010, from http://www.who.int/hia/evidence/doh/en/

Young, T. K. (1998). *Population health: Concepts and methods.* New York: Oxford University Press.

2

Origins of Public Health

INTRODUCTION

How is public health practiced in the United States today? To examine this issue, we will first discuss the origins of public health in the Industrial Revolution of the 18th and 19th centuries. Early industrialization, and the human misery that was its consequence, set the stage for public health as a professional field—its sense of identity, organization, goals, methods, and "sensibility." In previous eras, societies have practiced "public health"; in that, they may have provided healthful conditions for their people. The Romans built the great aqueducts, for instance, to bring clean water to the city. The Venetians during the 17th and 18th centuries controlled plague through public measures including surveillance and control of travel:

> During the 17th and 18th centuries, measures were taken by the Venetian administration to combat plague on the Ionian Islands. At that time, although the scientific basis of plague was unknown, the Venetians recognized its infectious nature and successfully decreased its spread by implementing an information network. Additionally, by activating a system of inspection that involved establishing garrisons along the coasts, the Venetians were able to control all local movements in plague-infested areas, which were immediately isolated. In contrast, the neighboring coast of mainland Greece, which was under Ottoman rule, was a plague-endemic area during the same period. . . . even in the absence of scientific knowledge, close observation and social and political measures can effectively restrain infectious outbreaks to the point of disappearance. (Konstantinidou, Mantadakis, Falagas, Sardi, & Samonis, 2009 p. 39)

However, modern public health aims in addition to prevent and control disease and injury in populations—a goal in evidence throughout human history—the aspiration for social justice. This public health "sensibility" is intolerant of disparities in health between those who have wealth, power, and status, and those who do not (Krieger & Birn, 1998). This "sensibility"

49

was clearly apparent in the early period of the Industrial Revolution and lead to the great achievements that we ascribe to public health in the 19th and 20th centuries and strive to emulate today.

Classification of Health Problems

Before considering the origins of modern public health, we need a classification scheme for health problems. We can consider health problems to be of two broad types: diseases and injuries. Diseases can be classified as infectious or noninfectious, with infectious diseases caused by pathogenic microorganisms— bacteria, viruses, fungi, multicellular parasites, and prions—that can be transmitted from person to person or from other species to persons. The term communicable disease is used interchangeably with infectious disease, as a result. Examples of infectious diseases are tuberculosis, plague, cholera, influenza, and human immunodeficiency virus (HIV). Noninfectious diseases are those that are not caused by a pathogenic microbe, but by factors that are not communicable or contagious such as environmental exposures to toxins, nutritional deficiencies, health behaviors, and genetic inheritance. They include dietary and autoimmune conditions; hereditary diseases such as hemophilia; diabetes; cardiovascular disease; and cancer. Mental health conditions such as depression, anxiety, and others are noninfectious. Noninfectious diseases are sometimes referred to as chronic diseases. However, the concept of chronic and acute may be applied to either infectious or noninfectious diseases. For example, HIV infection has become a chronic condition, at least in developed countries such as the United States, and nutritional deficiency diseases, once diagnosed, can be acute; that is, curable without lingering or permanent effects.

Injuries are the other broad category of health problems. A useful classification of injuries for public health practice is intentional and unintentional. Intentional injuries are self-inflicted such as suicide or inflicted by a person or persons on others such as homicide. Intentional injuries may result in death or morbidity. Domestic violence, child abuse, and elder abuse are intentional injuries. Unintentional or accidental injuries, again, can be self-inflicted or inflicted by others and result in mortality or morbidity. The most common unintentional injuries result from motor vehicle crashes, but injuries in the home and workplace are sites of a great many unintentional injuries including burns, falls, drownings, poisonings, and lacerations.

Distinguishing between diseases and injuries, infectious and non-infectious diseases, and intentional and unintentional injuries facilitates an understanding of the causes of health problems, and therefore, strategies to prevent them.

LIFE DURING THE INDUSTRIAL REVOLUTION

The history of modern public health in the United States and elsewhere has its roots in the Industrial Revolution. The exemplar is Britain. During industrialization, cities grew rapidly as factories replaced the domestic system of production, beginning with textiles. The poor living and working conditions in the burgeoning industrial cities, where infectious diseases were prevalent and frequently epidemic, are well documented. Housing was crowded, sanitation was grossly inadequate, clean water was scarce, and a healthful diet was beyond the means of most people. Work consisted of long days in unsafe and poorly ventilated factories, often exposed to toxic substances. Following are descriptions of housing and factory conditions in Britain, where industrialization first took root and had a profound effect on public health everywhere, including the United States, particularly in the development of the public health "sensibility."

Living Conditions

In the 1800s, London was an unsavory place to live for most people. The smells of raw sewage, horse and cattle manure, slaughter houses, unwashed bodies, and coal fires filled the air. Fog from the smoke of these fires made breathing difficult. Housing was cramped, often airless, and without a clean water supply or sanitary disposal of garbage and sewage. Diet was poor. On housing in London, Dr. Vinen, a medical officer of health, reported in 1856 on the living conditions typical of the day:

> In one small miserably dirty dilapidated room, occupied by a man, his wife and four children, in which they live day and night, was a child in its coffin that had died of measles eleven days before and, although decomposition was going on, it had not even been fastened down. The excuse made for its not having been buried before was that burials by the parish did not take place unless there were more than one to convey away at a time . . . In another miserable apartment scarce seven feet wide lived five persons and in which there was not one atom of furniture of any kind; the room contained nothing but a heap of filthy rags on the floor . . . The front door is never closed day or night and in consequence the staircase and landing form a nightly resort for thieves and prostitutes, where every kind of nuisance is committed . . . There are two yards at the back of this house, in each of which is an open privy; one of them is so abominably filthy and emitted a smell so foul that I was almost overpowered. (Spartacus Educational, 2010f, Dr. Vinen, para. 1)

Factory Life

Factories of the period were grim places to work. Many interviews with adult and child laborers testify to the conditions that often led to injury, permanent disability, and disease. Long hours, little rest, poor ventilation, exposure to dangerous equipment and chemicals, and harsh enforcement of workplace rules were the norm. There is no substitute for the words of those who experienced the conditions themselves.

John Birley, a worker in a 19th century mill, was interviewed by *The Ashton Chronicle* in 1849 about his life in Cressbrook Mill, where he began working when he was about 7 years old (Spartacus Educational, 2010e):

> Our regular time was from five in the morning till nine or ten at night; and on Saturday, till eleven, and often twelve o'clock at night, and then we were sent to clean the machinery on the Sunday. No time was allowed for break-fast and no sitting for dinner and no time for tea. We went to the mill at five o'clock and worked till about eight or nine when they brought us our breakfast, which consisted of water-porridge, with oatcake in it and onions to flavour it. Dinner consisted of Derbyshire oatcakes cut into four pieces, and ranged into two stacks. One was buttered and the other treacled. By the side of the oatcake were cans of milk. We drank the milk and with the oatcake in our hand, we went back to work without sitting down. (John Birley, para. 1)

A child who was interviewed by Michael Sadler's Parliamentary Committee in1832 gave the following account of how factory hours were kept (Spartacus Educational, 2010i):

> I worked at Mr. Braid's Mill at Duntruin. We worked as long as we could see. I could not say at what hour we stopped. There was no clock in the mill. There was nobody but the master and the master's son had a watch and so we did not know the time. The operatives were not permitted to have a watch. There was one man who had a watch but it was taken from him because he told the men the time. (James Patterson, para. 1)

Factory accidents were a major safety problem.

> Unguarded machinery was a major problem for children working in factories. One hospital reported that every year it treated nearly a thousand people for wounds and mutilations caused by machines in factories. A report commis-sioned by the House of Commons in 1832 said that: "there are factories, no means few in number, nor confined to the smaller mills, in which serious

accidents are continually occurring, and in which, notwithstanding, dangerous parts of the machinery are allowed to remain unfenced." The report added that the workers were often "abandoned from the moment that an accident occurs; their wages are stopped, no medical attendance is provided, and whatever the extent of the injury, no compensation is afforded." In 1842 a German visitor noted that he had seen so many people in the streets of Manchester without arms and legs that it was like "living in the midst of the army just returned from a campaign." (Spartacus Educational, 2010c, paras. 1–3)

Poorly ventilated factory buildings were another serious problem (Spartacus Educational, 2010d).

A report published in July 1833 stated that most factories were "dirty; low-roofed; ill-ventilated; ill-drained; no conveniences for washing or dressing; no contrivance for carrying off dust and other effluvia."

Sir Anthony Carlile, a doctor at Westminster Hospital visited some textile mills in 1832. He later gave evidence to the House of Commons on the dangers that factory pollution was causing for the young people working in factories: "labour is undergone in an atmosphere heated to a temperature of 70 to 80 and upwards." He pointed out that going from a "very hot room into damp cold air will inevitably produce inflammations of the lungs."

Doctors were also concerned about the "dust from flax and the flue from cotton" in the air that the young workers were breathing in. Dr. Charles Aston Key told Michael Sadler that this "impure air breathed for a great length of time must be productive of disease, or exceedingly weaken the body." Dr. Thomas Young who studied textile workers in Bolton reported that factory pollution was causing major health problems.

Most young workers complained of feeling sick during their first few weeks of working in a factory. Robert Blincoe said he felt that the dust and flue was suffocating him. This initial reaction to factory pollution became known as *mill fever*. Symptoms included sickness and headaches. The dust and floating cotton fibre in the atmosphere was a major factor in the high incidence of tuberculosis, bronchitis, asthma and byssinosis[1] amongst cotton workers. (paras. 1–5)

---

[1] Byssinosis is a lung disease caused by breathing cotton dust or dusts from other fibers such as flax, hemp, or sisal.

Child Labor

Child labor in textile factories and coal mines was perhaps the most appalling fact of the early period of industrialization. Following are interviews with two children about their experiences in the textile factories of London. The interviews were conducted for government investigations into the working conditions of children (Spartacus Educational, 2010b). Again, there is no substitute for the words of those who experienced these conditions themselves.

Charles Aberdeen was interviewed by Michael Sadler and his House of Commons Committee on 23rd July, 1832.
Question: How young have you known children go into silk mills.
Answer: I have known three at six; but very few at that age.
Question: What were your hours of labour?
Answer: From six in the morning till seven at night.
Question: Was it found necessary to beat children to keep them up to their employment?
Answer: Certainly.
Question: Did the beating increase towards evening?
Answer: Their strength relaxes more towards the evening; they get tired, and they twist themselves about on their legs, and stand on the sides of their feet.
Question: As an overlooker did you stimulate them to labour by severity?
Answer: Certainly, my employer always considered this indispensable.
Question: Did you not find it very irksome to your feelings, to have to take those means of urging the children to the work?
Answer: Extremely so; I have been compelled to urge them on to work when I knew they could not bear it; but I was obliged to make them strain every nerve to do the work, and I can say I have been disgusted with myself and with my situation; I felt myself degraded and reduced to the level of a slave-driver in such cases.
Question: Is not tying the broken ends, or piecing, an employment that requires great activity.
Answer: Yes.

Question: Does not the material often cut the hands of those poor children?

Answer: Frequently; but some more than others. I have seen them stand at their work, with their hands cut, till the blood has been running down to the ends of their fingers.

Question: Is there more work required of the children than there used to be when you first knew the business?

Answer: Yes; on account of the competition which exists between masters. One undersells the other; consequently the master endeavours to get an equal quantity of work done for less money. (Spartacus Educational, 2010b, Factory Workers section, William Rastrick)

Eliza Marshall was born in Doncaster in 1815. At the age of nine her family moved to Leeds where she found work at a local textile factory. Eliza was interviewed by Michael Sadler and his House of Commons Committee on 26th May, 1832.

Question: What was your hours of work?

Answer: When I first went to the mill we worked for six in the morning till seven in the evening. After a time we began at five in the morning, and worked till ten at night.

Question: Were you very much fatigued by that length of labour?

Answer: Yes.

Question: Did they beat you?

Answer: When I was younger they used to do it often.

Question: Did the labour affect your limbs?

Answer: Yes, when we worked over-hours I was worse by a great deal; I had stuff to rub my knees; and I used to rub my joints a quarter of an hour, and sometimes an hour or two.

Question: Were you straight before that?

Answer: Yes, I was; my master knows that well enough; and when I have asked for my wages, he said that I could not run about as I had been used to do.

Question: Are you crooked now?

Answer: Yes, I have an iron on my leg; my knee is contracted.

Question: Have the surgeons in the Infirmary told you by what your deformity was occasioned?

Answer: Yes, one of them said it was by standing; the marrow is dried out of the bone, so that there is no natural strength in it.
Question: You were quite straight till you had to labour so long in those mills?
Answer: Yes, I was as straight as anyone. (Spartacus Educational, 2010b, Factory Workers section, Eliza Marshall)

Following is an interview with a man who became a piecer in a mill as a child (Spartacus Educational, 2010h):

When I achieved the manly age of ten I obtained half-time employment at Dowry Mill as a "little piecer." . . . The noise was what impressed me most. Clatter, rattle, bang, the swish of thrusting levers and the crowding of hundreds of men, women and children at their work. Long rows of huge spinning-frames, with thousands of whirling spindles, slid forward several feet, paused and then slid smoothly back again, continuing the process unceasingly hour after hour while cotton became yarn and yarn changed to weaving material. Often the threads on the spindles broke as they were stretched and twisted and spun. These broken ends had to be instantly repaired; the piecer ran forward and joined them swiftly, with a deft touch that is an art of its own. I remember no golden summers, no triumphs at games and sports, no tramps through dark woods or over shadow-racing hills. Only meals at which there never seemed to be enough food, dreary journeys through smoke-fouled streets, in mornings when I nodded with tiredness and in evenings when my legs trembled under me from exhaustion. (J. R. Clynes, paras. 1–4)

Finally, here is another account of childhood spent in a mill from a young man interviewed by William Dodd in 1842 (Spartacus Educational, 2010a):

I am about twenty-five years old. I have been a piecer at Mr. Cousen's worsted mill, I have worked nowhere else. I commenced working in a worsted mill at nine years of age. Our hours of labour were from six in the morning to seven and eight at night, with thirty minutes off at noon for dinner. We had no time for breakfast or drinking. The children conceive it to be a very great mischief; to be kept so long in labour; and I believe their parents would be very glad if it was not so. I found it very hard and laborious employment. I had 2s. per week at first. We had to stoop, to bend our bodies and our legs.

I was a healthy and strong boy, when I first went to the mill. When I was about eight years old, I could walk from Leeds to Bradford (ten miles) without any pain or difficulty, and with a little fatigue; now I cannot stand without crutches! I cannot walk at all! Perhaps I might creep up stairs. I go up stairs backwards every night! I found my limbs begin to fail, after I had been working about a year. It came on with great pain in my legs and knees. I am very much fatigued towards the end of the day. I cannot work in the mill now.

The overlooker beat me up to my work! I have been beaten till I was black and blue and I have had my ears torn! Once I was very ill with it. He beat me then, because I mixed a few empty bobbins, not having any place to put them in separate. we were beaten most at the latter end of the day, when we grew tired and fatigued. The highest wages I ever had in the factory, were 5s. 6d. per week.

My mother is dead; my father was obliged to send me to the mill, in order to keep me. I had to attend at the mill after my limbs began to fail. I could not then do as well as I could before. I had one shilling a week taken off my wages. I had lost several inches in height. I had frequently to stand thirteen and fourteen hours a day, and to be continually engaged. I was perfectly straight before I entered on this labour.

Other boys were deformed in the same way. A good many boys suffered in their health, in consequence of the severity of their work. I am sure this pain, and grievous deformity, came from my long hours of labour. My father, and my friends, believe so to. It is the opinion of all the medical men who have seen me. (Benjamin Gomersal, paras. 1–5)

Health Problems of the Times

The squalid and unsafe living and working conditions in industrialized cities of 19th century Britain led to infectious disease outbreaks and epidemics, especially among the poor. Children were at most risk of death from infectious disease. The appalling working and living conditions of the poor and working classes during the industrialization of Europe, the United States, and similar countries also had a profound impact on the risk of injuries and noninfectious diseases. Lack of attention to safety in the workplace was a major cause of injuries and disabilities. In addition, the wages that families had for necessities were often unable to pay for healthful foods, and nutritional deficiency diseases were common.

MODERN PUBLIC HEALTH IS BORN

Public Outcry

The living and working conditions for the ordinary person during this period provoked a progressive outcry for change. Child labor was especially galvanizing. Work in the factories and coal mines was long, hard, and dirty for all laborers. However, protection of children and women became a cause for many progressive leaders of the time. The following excerpt from a poem written in 1836 by Caroline Sheridan Norton (anonymous at the time) is an example of the sentiments held by many persons about child labor practices in Britain at the time (Norton, 1836). Prefacing the poem, which was meant to be presented in Parliament, the author stated the following:

The abuses even, of such a business, must be cautiously dealt with; lest, in eradicating them, we shake or disorder the whole fabric. We admit, however, that the case of CHILDREN employed in the Cotton Factories is one of those that call fairly for legislative regulation (para. 1):

These then are his Companions: he, too young
To share their base and saddening merriment,
Sits by: his little head in silence hung;
His limbs cramped up; his body weakly bent;
Toiling obedient, till long hours so spent
Produce Exhaustion's slumber, dull and deep.
The Watcher's stroke,–bold–sudden–violent,–
Urges him from that lethargy of sleep,
And bids him wake to Life,–to labour and to weep!
But the day hath its End. Forth then he hies
With jaded, faltering step, and brow of pain;
Creeps to that shed,–his HOME,–where happy lies
The sleeping babe that cannot toil for Gain;
Where his remorseful Mother tempts in vain
With the best portion of their frugal fare:
Too sick to eat–too weary to complain–
He turns him idly from the untasted share,
Slumbering sinks down unfed, and mocks her useless care. (Norton,
1836, A Voice from the Factories, paras. 48–49)

The author added about the poem:

I will only add, that I have in *no* instance overcharged or exaggerated, by poetical fictions, the picture drawn by the Commissioners appointed to inquire into this subject. I have strictly adhered to the printed Reports; to that which I believe to be the melancholy truth; and that which I have, in some instances, myself had an opportunity of witnessing.

I earnestly hope I shall live to see this evil abolished. There will be delay–there will be opposition: such has ever been the case with all questions involving interests, and more especially *[Page ix]* where the preponderating interest has been on the side of the existing abuse. Yet, as the noble-hearted and compassionate Howard became immortally connected with the removal of the abuses which for centuries disgraced our prison discipline; as the perseverance of Wilberforce created the dawn of the long-delayed emancipation of the negroes;–so, my Lord, I trust to see *your* name enrolled with the names of these great and good men, as the Liberator and Defender of those helpless beings, on whom are inflicted many of the evils both of slavery and imprisonment, without the odium of either. (Norton, 1836, Dedicated to the Right Honourable Lord Ashley, paras. 7–8)

Another famous speech, given by Lord Byron before the House of Lords in 1812, defended the Luddites who had engaged in violence provoked by the loss of employment due to the industrialization of textile manufacture:

During the short time I recently passed in Nottingham, not twelve hours elapsed without some fresh act of violence; and on that day I left the county I was informed that forty Frames had been broken the preceding evening, as usual, without resistance and without detection.

Such was the state of that county, and such I have reason to believe it to be at this moment. But whilst these outrages must be admitted to exist to an alarming extent, it cannot be denied that they have arisen from circumstances of the most unparalleled distress: the perseverance of these miserable men in their proceedings, tends to prove that nothing but absolute want could have driven a large, and once honest and industrious, body of the people, into the commission of excesses so hazardous to themselves, their families, and the community.

They were not ashamed to beg, but there was none to relieve them: their own means of subsistence were cut off, all other employment preoccupied; and their excesses, however to be deplored and condemned, can hardly be subject to surprise.

As the sword is the worst argument than can be used, so should it be the last. In this instance it has been the first; but providentially as yet only in the scabbard. The present measure will, indeed, pluck it from the sheath; yet had proper meetings been held in the earlier stages of these riots, had the grievances of these men and their masters (for they also had their grievances) been fairly weighed and justly examined, I do think that means might have been devised to restore these workmen to their avocations, and tranquillity [*sic*] to the country. (Spartacus Educational, 2010g, Lord Byron, paras. 1–4)

Public Response to Infectious Disease Outbreaks

The high rate of infectious diseases in the industrializing British cities, including the cholera outbreaks of 1817, 1849, and 1854 in London, brought about a public health response. The 1854 outbreak was the one for which John Snow identified the *broad street pump* as the cause, and although it was not known that the bacteria *Vibrio cholera* was present in the water gathered at the pump, it was evident from Snow's epidemiological investigation that it was the source of the disease outbreak.

The method used to address the problem of infectious diseases in Britain and other industrializing countries during the 1800s was environmental engineering—the archetypical primary prevention strategy—which modified the environment for all persons at risk. Although the microbial agents of infectious diseases were unknown at the time, public health engineering programs in the 1800s provided clean water and removal of sewage and garbage for the effort to reduce the problem of infectious disease outbreaks.

By the 1800s, people began to understand that unsanitary living conditions and water contamination contributed to disease epidemics. This new awareness prompted major cities to take measures to control waste and garbage. In the mid-1850s, Chicago built the first major sewage system in the United States to treat wastewater. Soon, many other U.S. cities followed Chicago's lead. (National Oceanic and Atmospheric Administration [NOAA], 2010, para. 2)

Later in the century, the discoveries that led to vaccines and antimicrobial therapies, such as penicillin, resulted in further reduction in the threat of infectious diseases.

Public Response to Injuries and Noninfectious Diseases

The working conditions that led to injury and disability during the Industrial Revolution in Britain also produced a public response. Many people, as we have seen, wished to see an end to the abuse of workers under the factory system. With respect to child labor, the public response was an investigation of conditions by officials in the government and eventual passage of legislation. In 1831, the Sadler Committee, chaired by Michael Thomas Sadler, was charged with investigating conditions of child labor in cotton and linen factories. In 1833, a parliamentary commission was appointed to investigate working conditions in other textile industries. In 1842, a committee chaired by Lord Ashley investigated conditions in coal mines. Following is a summary of the laws enacted in Britain from 1819 to 1891 to protect workers, particularly children:

1819—Factory Act: Limits working days for children in cotton mills to 12 hours. Children younger than the age of 9 should not be employed, but magistrates did not enforce this.

In 1833, the government passed a Factory Act to improve conditions for children working in factories. Young children were working very long hours in workplaces where conditions were often terrible. The basic act was as follows:

1. There should be no child workers younger than 9 years of age.
2. Employers must have a medical or age certificate for child workers.
3. Children between the ages of 9 and 13 to work no more than 9 hours a day.
4. Children between the ages of 13 and 18 to work no more than 12 hours a day.
5. Children are not to work at night.
6. There should be two hours schooling each day for children.
7. Four factory inspectors must be appointed to enforce the law throughout the whole of the country.

However, the passing of this Act did not mean that overnight, the mistreatment of children stopped.

1842—Mines Act: Women and girls, and boys younger than the age of 10, were not allowed to work underground. Boys younger than the age of 15 were not allowed to work on machinery.
1844—Factory Act: Children younger than 13 years to work no more than 6.5 hours a day. Women and children aged 13–18 to work no more than 12 hours a day.
1847—Factory Act: Limits women and children younger than 18 years to 58-hour working week.
1850—Factory Act: Establishes standard working day.
1860—Mines Act: Boys younger than 12 years are not allowed underground unless they could read and write.
1875—Act passed that required all chimney sweeps to be licensed. Licensees were issued only to sweeps not using climbing boys.
1878—Factory and Workshops Act: Employment of children younger than 10 years is banned. Regulations of control safety, ventilation, and meals.
1891—Factory Act made the requirements for fencing machinery more stringent. Under the heading "Conditions of Employment," two considerable additions were included to previous legislation. The first is the prohibition on employers to employ women within 4 weeks after confinement; the second is the raising of minimum age at which a child can be set to work from 10 to 11 years old (Ward, 2010).

Public response to the health problems brought about by the Industrial Revolution—both diseases and injuries—laid the foundation for public health as a professional field in Britain and other industrializing countries in Europe and the Americas. From the cauldron, which was the industrializing cities of the 19th century, came what have become permanent public health commitments to workplace safety, child and maternal health, safe and healthful housing conditions, sanitary disposal of waste, and a safe and nutritious food supply. Concern for "vulnerable" populations and the desire to reduce health disparities and increase health equity are at the heart of many, if not most public health goals and activities today. This "public health sensibility" also, it can be argued, arose among progressive elites in response to the inequities and hardships of the poor and working people during the Industrial Revolution.

SUCCESS OF PUBLIC HEALTH MEASURES

Infectious diseases were the major cause of morbidity and mortality in Britain, as well as the rest of the world, through the end of the 19th century. Common infectious diseases included smallpox, chicken pox, cholera, malaria, diphtheria, and scarlet fever. Some diseases were not fatal, but others were responsible for most of the deaths at the turn of the century. Some, such as smallpox, could be disfiguring for life.

Environmental engineering projects that were begun in the 1800s resulted in improved control of infectious diseases and some of the greatest successes of public health. Later, advancements in the microscope and microbiology led to effective treatments for infectious diseases that in the past were death sentences. They also led to the development of vaccines to prevent infectious diseases from occurring.

Control of infectious diseases has resulted from clean water and improved sanitation. Infections such as typhoid and cholera transmitted by contaminated water, a major cause of illness and death early in the 20th century, have been reduced dramatically by improved sanitation. In addition, the discovery of antimicrobial therapy has been critical to successful public health efforts to control infections such as tuberculosis and sexually transmitted diseases (STDs). (Centers for Disease Control and Prevention [CDC], 1999)

These developments—primary prevention through sanitary engineering and vaccines, and secondary prevention through antibiotics and other antimicrobial drugs—changed dramatically the reasons people died in the 20th century, as well as their age of death. Thus, the success of public health efforts with regard to infectious diseases—through primary and secondary prevention—is evident in changes in the leading causes of death and in life expectancy since the 19th century.

Information about the causes of death is obtained from death certificates and how they are coded and compiled:

For the purpose of national mortality statistics, every death is attributed to one underlying condition, based on information reported on the death certificate and using the international rules for selecting the underlying cause of death from the conditions stated on the certificate. The underlying cause is defined by the World Health Organization (WHO) as "the disease or injury that initiated the train of events leading directly to death, or the circumstances of the accident or violence that produced the fatal injury." Generally, more medical information is reported on death certificates than is directly reflected in the underlying cause of death. Conditions that are not selected as underlying cause of death constitute the nonunderlying causes of death, also known as multiple cause of death. . . . Selected causes of death of public health and medical importance are compiled into tabulation lists and are ranked according to the number of deaths assigned to these causes. The top-ranking causes determine the leading causes of death. (National Center for Health Statistics [NCHS], 2010b, p. 502).

The United States is a good example of how the causes of death have changed since the era of infectious diseases. The leading causes of death are considerably different now than in 1900. The leading causes of death in 1900 in the United States (see Table 2.1) reflect the significance of infectious diseases. Deaths from infectious diseases were continuing to decline in 1900, but were still major health threats. At the turn of the century, the first three causes of death were infectious diseases—pneumonia and influenza; tuberculosis; diarrhea and enteritis; and ulceration of the intestines. These, along with diphtheria, accounted for 34% of all deaths at that time.

Now, infectious diseases are far less important causes of death than noninfectious diseases including heart, cerebrovascular, and respiratory diseases, cancer, and diabetes (see Table 2.2). The only infectious diseases among the 10 leading

TABLE 2.1   Leading Causes of Death: United States, 1900

Cause of Death	Number of Deaths	% of All Deaths
All causes	343,217	100
Pneumonia (all forms) and influenza	40,362	11.76
Tuberculosis (all forms)	38,820	11.31
Diarrhea, enteritis, and ulceration of the intestines	28,491	8.30
Diseases of the heart	27,427	7.99
Intracranial lesions of vascular origin (stroke)	21,353	6.22
Nephritis (all forms)	17,699	5.16
All accidents	14,429	4.20
Cancer and other malignant tumors	12,769	3.72
Senility	10,015	2.92
Diphtheria	8,056	2.35

Note: National Center for Health Statistics (NCHS), 2010a.

TABLE 2.2   **Leading Causes of Death: United States, 2006**

Cause of Death	Number of Deaths	% of All Deaths
All causes	2,426,264	100
Diseases of the heart	631,636	26.03
Malignant neoplasm	559,888	23.08
Cerebrovascular diseases	137,119	5.65
Chronic lower respiratory diseases	124,583	5.13
Unintentional injury	121,599	5.01
Diabetes mellitus	72,449	2.99
Alzheimer's disease	72,432	2.99
Influenza and pneumonia	56,326	2.32
Nephritis, nephritic syndrome and nephrosis	45,344	1.87
Septicemia	34,234	1.41

Source: National Center for Health Statistics (NCHS), 2010b.

causes of death—influenza and pneumonia, and septicemia—account for only 4% of all deaths. Further, most pneumonia and septicemia deaths now occur during hospitalizations at the end of life, not among the young.

However, it should be noted that infectious diseases remain a problem, even though noninfectious diseases predominate now. New infectious diseases have emerged, as for example, HIV, which has had an effect on mortality among young people. Old infectious diseases have become resistant to standard treatments. For example, methicillin-resistant *Staphylococcus aureus* (MRSA), both community- and hospital-acquired, is a great concern. As the CDC reports: "MRSA can be fatal. In 1974, MRSA infections accounted for 2% of the total number of staph infections; in 1995 it was 22%; in 2004 it was 63%. CDC estimated that 94,360 invasive MRSA infections occurred in the United States in 2005; 18,650 of these were associated with death" (CDC, 2010).

Life expectancy also reflects success in controlling infectious disease. "Life expectancy is a measure often used to gauge the overall health of a population. As a summary measure of mortality, life expectancy represents the average number of years of life that could be expected if current death rates were to remain constant. Shifts in life expectancy are often used to describe trends in mortality. Life expectancy at birth is strongly influenced by infant and child mortality. Life expectancy later in life reflects death rates at or above a given age and is independent of the effect of mortality at younger ages. (NCHS, 2010b, p. 44)

TABLE 2.3   Life Expectancy by Age: Death Registration States, 1900–1902 to 1909–1911, and United States, 1929–1931 to 2006

Age and Race	Average Number of Years of Life Remaining						
	1900–1902	1909–1911	1929–1931	1949–1951	1969–1971	1989–1991	2006
All races							
0	49.24	51.49	59.20	68.07	70.75	75.37	77.7
1	55.20	57.11	61.94	69.16	71.19	75.08	77.2
5	54.98	56.21	59.29	65.54	67.43	71.22	73.3
10	51.14	52.15	54.84	60.74	62.57	66.29	68.4
20	42.79	43.53	45.94	51.20	53.00	56.63	58.6
30	35.51	35.70	37.75	41.91	43.71	47.23	49.2
40	28.34	28.20	29.67	32.81	34.52	37.98	39.7
50	21.26	20.98	22.06	24.40	25.93	29.03	30.7
60	14.76	14.42	15.24	17.04	18.34	20.90	22.4
70	9.30	9.11	9.58	10.92	12.00	13.96	14.9
80	5.30	5.25	5.50	6.34	7.10	8.40	8.7

Source: Arias, 2010.

The control of infectious diseases, which began with the sanitary and housing improvements in the 1800s and ended with microbial treatments and vaccines in the late 19th and 20th centuries, was a major cause of increased life expectancy in the first half of the 20th century. This is particularly true for young people who were most at risk for death from diseases such as cholera, typhoid, diphtheria, and other infections. As an example, Table 2.3 contains the life expectancies for all people from 1900 through 2006 in the United States (Arias, 2010).[2] Between 1900 and 2006, children at birth and at the age of 1 year experienced a 58% and 40% increase in life expectancy, respectively, largely in the first half of the century. About 65% and 62%, respectively, of the overall increase for these ages came prior to 1951.

In contrast, life expectancy for adults 60 years and older increased more after 1951. People 60, 70, and 80 years old experienced an increase in life expectancy between 1900 and 2006 of 52%, 60%, and 64%, respectively. However, only about 28% of this increase for each age group occurred prior

[2] Alaska and Hawaii included beginning in 1959. For decennial periods prior to 1929–1931, data are for groups of registration states as follows: 1900–1902 and 1909–1911, 10 states and the District of Columbia (D.C.); 1919–1921, 34 states and D.C. Beginning 1970 excludes deaths of nonresidents of the United States.

to 1951. In the age of the great infectious disease epidemics, the control measures had only small effects on those who survived childhood.

Public health has had many accomplishments since its successes in infectious disease control in the 19th and early 20th centuries. The CDC (1999) has developed a list of the 10 greatest public health achievements in the United States since 1900. The average lifespan has increased by more than 30 years in the United States, and the CDC attributes 25 years of this gain to public health measures. The 10 achievements selected by the CDC were "based on the opportunity for prevention and the impact on death, illness, and disability" (p. 241). They are listed as follows:

10 Great Public Health Achievements—United States, 1900–1999

1. *Vaccination.* Vaccination has resulted in eradication of smallpox; elimination of poliomyelitis in the Americas; and control of measles, rubella, tetanus, diphtheria, Haemophilus influenza type b, and other infectious diseases in the United States and other parts of the world.
2. *Motor vehicle safety.* Improvements in motor vehicle safety have resulted from engineering efforts to make both vehicles and highways safer, and from successful efforts to change personal behavior (e.g., increased use of safety belts, child safety seats, and motorcycle helmets, and decreased drinking and driving). These efforts have contributed to large reductions in motor vehicle–related deaths.
3. *Safer workplaces.* Work-related health problems such as coal workers' pneumoconiosis (black lung) and silicosis—common at the beginning of the century—have come under better control. Severe injuries and deaths related to mining, manufacturing, construction, and transportation also have decreased; since 1980, safer workplaces have resulted in a reduction of approximately 40% in the rate of fatal occupational injuries.
4. *Control of infectious diseases.* Control of infectious diseases has resulted from clean water and improved sanitation. Infections such as typhoid and cholera transmitted by contaminated water, a major cause of illness and death early in the 20th century, have been reduced dramatically by improved sanitation. In addition,

the discovery of antimicrobial therapy has been critical to successful public health efforts to control infections such as tuberculosis and sexually transmitted diseases (STDs).

5. *Decline in deaths from coronary heart disease and stroke.* Decline in deaths from coronary heart disease and stroke have resulted from risk-factor modification such as smoking cessation and blood pressure control coupled with improved access to early detection and better treatment. Since 1972, death rates for coronary heart disease have decreased 51%.

6. *Safer and healthier foods.* Since 1900, safer and healthier foods have resulted from decreases in microbial contamination and increases in nutritional content. Identifying essential micronutrients and establishing food-fortification programs have almost eliminated major nutritional deficiency diseases such as rickets, goiter, and pellagra in the United States.

7. *Healthier mothers and babies.* Healthier mothers and babies have resulted from better hygiene and nutrition, availability of antibiotics, greater access to health care, and technologic advances in maternal and neonatal medicine. Since 1900, infant mortality has decreased 90%, and maternal mortality has decreased 99%.

8. *Family planning.* Access to family planning and contraceptive services has altered social and economic roles of women. Family planning has provided health benefits such as smaller family size and longer interval between the birth of children; increased opportunities for preconceptional counseling and screening; fewer infant, child, and maternal deaths; and the use of barrier contraceptives to prevent pregnancy and transmission of HIV and other STDs.

9. *Fluoridation of drinking water.* Fluoridation of drinking water began in 1945, and in 1999 reached an estimated 144 million persons in the United States. Fluoridation safely and inexpensively benefits both children and adults by effectively preventing tooth decay, regardless of socioeconomic status or access to care. Fluoridation has played an important role in the reductions in tooth decay (40%–70% in children) and of tooth loss in adults (40%–60%).

10. *Recognition of tobacco use as a health hazard.* Recognition of to-bacco use as a health hazard and subsequent public health an-tismoking campaigns have resulted in changes in social norms to prevent initiation of tobacco use, promote cessation of use, and reduce exposure to environmental tobacco smoke. Since the 1964 Surgeon General's report on the health risks of smoking, the prevalence of smoking among adults has decreased, and millions of smoking-related deaths have been prevented.

Through the 19th century and into the 20th century, public health in the United States organized principally as a government effort and expanded its impact on the important health issues of the time. Public health practice continued to be influenced by the health and safety problems—infectious diseases and injuries—that predominated in the industrializing cities of Britain, the United States, and elsewhere during the Industrial Revolution, and the prevention measures that had been successful then. These included provision of clean water, sanitary removal of sewage and garbage, safe hous-ing, clean food supply, and safe workplaces. Development and provision of vaccines to prevent infectious diseases became an essential component of the public health toolkit. Public health also added initiatives in response to changing health needs, particularly the increase in noninfectious dis-eases such as heart, vascular, and respiratory diseases, diabetes, and cancer. Reducing health behaviors related to noninfectious disease risk including smoking, poor diet, and sedentary lifestyle became an integral part of public health practice. And as medical care became more effective, assuring avail-ability of hospital and physician services for those whose access was limited by poverty, geography, and health status became an important focus of pub-lic health efforts. The development of automobiles and the influence of mo-tor vehicle-related accidents on morbidity and mortality put this issue on the public health agenda as well. Emerging infectious diseases, particularly HIV and the antibiotic resistant strains of old infectious diseases have become important to public health. And threaded throughout the expanded public health agenda remains the drive to ensure that persons with the least power, influence, and resources have the opportunity to lead safe and healthy lives, just as the plight of child factory workers in the early 1800s moved British reformers to action on their behalf. The emphasis today on ending health disparities is testament to this enduring public health goal and the "public health sensibility" motivating it. This is not to say that public health has been entirely effective. Much has been done, but much remains to be done, as we will discuss in the final chapter.

REFERENCES

Arias, E. (2010). United States life tables, 2006. *National Vital Statistics Reports*, 58(21).

Centers for Disease Control and Prevention. (1999). Ten great public health achievements—United States, 1900–1999. *Morbidity and Mortality Weekly Report*, 48(12), 241–243.

Centers for Disease Control and Prevention. (2010). *Healthcare-associated methicillin resistant staphylococcus aureus (HA-MRSA)*. Retrieved July 10, 2010, from http://www.cdc.gov/ncidod/dhqp/ar_mrsa.html

Konstantinidou, K., Mantadakis, E., Falagas, M. E., Sardi, T., & Samonis, G. (2009). Venetian rule and control of plague epidemics on the Ionian Islands during 17th and 18th centuries. *Emerging Infectious Diseases, 15*(1), 39–43.

Krieger, N., & Birn, A. E. (1998). A vision of social justice as the foundation of public health: Commemorating 150 years of the spirit of 1848. *American Journal of Public Health, 88*(11), 1603–1606.

National Center for Health Statistics. (2010a). *Leading causes of death, 1900–1998*. Retrieved July 13, 2010, from http://cdc.gov/nchs/data/dvs/lead1900_98.pdf

National Center for Health Statistics. (2010b). Table 28. *Health United States 2009 with special feature on medical technology*. Hyattsville, MD.

National Oceanic and Atmospheric Administration. (2010). *Nonpoint source pollution: A brief history of pollution*. Retrieved July 13, 2010, from http://oceanservice.noaa.gov/education/kits/pollution/02history.html

Norton, C. S. (1836). *A voice from the factories*. Retrieved July 10, 2010, from http://digital.library.upenn.edu/women/norton/avftf/avftf.html

Pike, E. R. (1966). *Hard times: Human documents of the industrial revolution*. New York: Praeger.

Spartacus Educational. (2010a). *Benjamin Gomersal*. Retrieved July 10, 2010, from http://www.spartacus.schoolnet.co.uk/IRgomersal.htm

Spartacus Educational. (2010b). *Child labour*. Retrieved July 14, 2010, from http://www.spartacus.schoolnet.co.uk/IRchild.htm

Spartacus Educational. (2010c). *Factory accidents*. Retrieved July 10, 2010, from http://www.spartacus.schoolnet.co.uk/IRaccidents.htm

Spartacus Educational. (2010d). *Factory pollution*. Retrieved July 10, 2010, from http://www.spartacus.schoolnet.co.uk/IRpollution.htm

Spartacus Educational. (2010e). *John Birley*. Retrieved July 10, 2010, from http://www.spartacus.schoolnet.co.uk/IRbirley.htm

Spartacus Educational. (2010f). *London*. Retrieved July 10, 2010, from http://www.spartacus.schoolnet.co.uk/ITlondon.htm

Spartacus Educational. (2010g). *Lord Byron*. Retrieved October 20, 2010, from http://www.spartacus.schoolnet.co.uk/PRbyron.htm

Spartacus Educational. (2010h). *Piecers*. Retrieved July 14, 2010, from http://www.spartacus.schoolnet.co.uk/IRpiecers.htm

Spartacus Educational. (2010i). *Working hours in factories*. Retrieved July 11, 2010, from http://www.spartacus.schoolnet.co.uk/IRtime.htm

Spartacus Educational. Lord Byron. Retrieved October 20, 2010 at http://www.spartacus.schoolnet.co.uk/PRbyron.htm

Thompson, E. P. (1964). *The making of the english working class*. New York: Pantheon Books.

Toynbee, A. (1957). *The industrial revolution*. Boston: Beacon Press.

Ward, P. (2010). *Children in the 1800's*. Retrieved July 14, 2010, from http://www.ourwardfamily.com/children_of_the_1800%27s.htm

3

Organization and Financing of Public Health

INTRODUCTION

The 2003 Institute of Medicine (IOM) report, *The Future of the Public's Health in the 21st Century*, emphasizes that public health extends beyond government and encompasses, "the efforts, science, art, and approaches used by all sectors of society (public, private, and civil society) to assure, maintain, protect, promote, and improve the health of the people"(Committee on Assuring the Health of the Public in the 21st Century, 2002, p. 20). The report defines six critical "actors" who are in a position to greatly affect health: communities, the health care delivery system, employers and business, the media, academia, and government.

Public health systems are commonly defined as "all public, private, and voluntary entities that contribute to the delivery of essential public health services within a jurisdiction." These systems are a network of entities with differing roles, relationships, and interactions. All of the entities within a public health system contribute to the health and well-being of the community or state. (Centers for Disease Control and Prevention [CDC], 2007, p. 3)

Other definitions of public health also emphasize the collaboration between the public and private sectors in the organization and activities of public health. Van Wave, Scutchfield, and Honoré (2010) assert that:

The public health system is defined as the collective resources, infrastructure, and effort of all public, private, and voluntary entities and their respective roles, relationships, and interactions that contribute to the delivery of essential public health services to the population within a jurisdiction (p. 284).

The CDC states: "The governmental public health agency—both at the state and local levels—is a major contributor and leader in the public health system, but these governmental agencies cannot provide the full spectrum of Essential

73

Services alone." (CDC, 2007, p. 4). The IOM (1988, p. 41) defines the public health system as the "activities undertaken within the formal structure of government and the associated efforts of private and voluntary organizations and individuals." Further, the IOM (2003) finds that a public health system is

> a complex network of individuals and organizations that have the potential to play critical roles in creating the conditions of health. They can act for health individually, but when they work together toward a health goal, they act as a system—a public health system (p. 28).

Although there is much to recommend this broader understanding of the public health system, it is also too extensive for an introduction. In this chapter, we will focus on the governmental public health system, with some attention to the private actors who frequently collaborate with it (e.g., academia, nonprofit health organizations, professional associations). The decision to focus on government is, in part, practical: taking an especially broad view of the public health "system," which encompasses a multitude of actors in all areas of society—largely without any formalized organization, relationships, or roles–renders it largely resistant to generalization, and as we will see, the governmental system is itself sufficiently complex all on its own. The decision is also, however, substantive:

> Governmental public health agencies constitute the backbone of the public health system and bear primary, legally mandated responsibility for assuring the delivery of essential public health services. Therefore, the role of government in assuring the nation's health is one that must be continued and sustained. (IOM, 2003, p. 27)

Government has a unique and special responsibility to promote public health. Governments also have the resources and legal authority to implement public health policies and focus public health missions that private actors generally lack. Accordingly, the focus of the discussion of the U.S. public health system will be on the government agencies, we should not lose sight of the fact that government frequently partners with other actors—academia, nongovernmental organizations (NGOs), professional associations, philanthropic organizations, the private health care delivery system, as well as business and media—in developing and delivering public health services.

> The integrating force for the public health system—the "glue"—is the official public health agency infrastructure. Only government has jurisdiction, the power to create and enforce laws, and the mandate to secure our

fundamental rights. In the United States, such duties rest within the governments of the fifty states and five territories, each of which has an organized public health unit that oversees the conduct of the government's public health programs and fulfills the roles that "cannot be properly delegated." (Tilson & Berkowitz, 2006, p. 904)

Government is also key because "public health" functions, at least in large part, are to provide for people who are not suitably or effectively provided for by the private sector.

Organization of Public Health System

The governmental public health system in the United States is comprised of several departments and agencies within the federal government, at least one state-level agency for every state and territory in the country, and approximately 2,800 local health agencies. Hundreds of thousands of public health workers staff these agencies (Association of State and Territorial Health Officials [ASTHO], 2008); U.S. Department of Health and Human Services [DHHS], 2009; National Association of County and City Health Officials [NACCHO, 2009]). Given our cognitive preference to find order in systems and our predispositions about the structure of organizations, it may be tempting to imagine from this rudimentary description that the U.S. public health system is a centralized, cohesive, hierarchically arranged organization in which the federal government sets policy and marshals resources, which it then distributes to the states, which in turn establish the infrastructure for implementation of those polices and provision of public health services to the population through local health departments, which then deliver them.

In truth, however, the governmental public health system in the United States is highly decentralized. The federal government has little direct control over state public health matters. States are generally responsible for their own public health systems, and in most circumstances, states delegate at least some of that authority to local political units—cities, towns, counties, and so forth—which set and implement their own public health policies. Rather than exercising *authority* over health matters in the United States, the federal government's role is primarily one of *influence*. This influence is broadly either of the "persuasive" variety, whereby research and recommendations conducted at the federal level inform the decisions of more local public health policymakers and actors, or of the "financial" variety, whereby the federal government provides financial support to state and local public health agencies, frequently on the condition that the funds be used in a particular manner. The limited authority the federal government does have is generally restricted to those issues that have been recognized as affecting commercial or business conditions across state lines. Thus, the U.S. government public health system is a highly complex system of discrete, often independent, decentralized, and varied agencies.

The decentralized and largely local character of the public health system is, in substantial part, a consequence of the legal, political, and historical context in which the public health system developed and operates. Largely, the organization of the public health system and the delivery of public health services can be traced to the principles of federalism governing the broader political and governmental organization of the United States (Turnock & Atchison, 2002). Under the U.S. federal system, sovereign power is shared between the federal government and the states, with certain powers delegated to the federal government exclusively, certain powers retained by the states exclusively, and some powers held by both the federal and state governments (subject to the limitations of federal supremacy). The 10th Amendment provides that any power not specifically delegated to the federal government in the Constitution be retained by the states. Among the powers the Constitution provides to the federal government is the power to tax and spend and to regulate interstate commerce. As will be discussed further, the activities of the federal government in support of public health generally derive from these powers. One power not specified in the Constitution, however, is the "police power"—the power to regulate and coerce persons for the benefit and welfare of society. Because it is not specified, it is among the plenary powers remaining with the states. It has long been recognized that the authority to regulate in the interest of public health derives from the police power ("The states of this Union may, in the exercise of their police powers, pass quarantine and health laws." *Passenger Cases*, [1849] Wayne, J., concurring). States, therefore, have primary authority for public health in the United States.

Consistent with federalism's placement of value on local self-determination, states often further pass on the police power, at least to some extent, to smaller and more local units of government (counties, cities, towns, etc.). This is true in the area of public health. Many states have delegated public health responsibilities to local governments or boards of health. Further, "home rule" statutes in 48 states authorize local governments, depending on factors including their size and class, to address public health issues directly through local laws (McCarty, Nelson, Hodge, & Gebbie, 2009). That public health concerns are considered under the federal system to be principally matters of local concern that is consistent with the historic emergence of public health practice and regulation in the United States. "Public health in the United States did not begin as a systematic, rational, centrally directed activity following a coherent plan but rather as a fitful, episodic, and necessity-driven response to immediate local threats" (Fee & Brown, 2002). Public health concerns—and health matters in general, for that matter—did not historically emerge as national issues, but as local ones, and the allocation of government responsibility—with state and the local government having primary responsibility for implementing public health regulations and delivery of public health services—reflects this.

That decentralized governmental public health authority and delivery in the United States is not necessarily problematic. Consistent with principals of federalism, theories of political economy suggest that superior public services may flow from decentralized governmental authority because the more local the government, the closer it is to the population it serves, making it more informed of and responsive to the needs of its population (Mays et al., 2006; Mays et al., 2007). However, in the last quarter century, the ability of the U.S. public health system to deliver the services required of it has come under scrutiny. The IOM's (1988) landmark report, *The Future of Public Health*, which is a frequent reference point for analysis and evaluation of the U.S. public health system, stimulated interest in assessment and improvement of the public health enterprise (Tilson & Berkowitz, 2006; Turnock & Atchison, 2002). The report noted that "[i]n recent years, there has been a growing sense that public health, as a profession, as a governmental activity, and as a commitment of society is neither clearly defined, adequately supported, nor fully understood" (IOM, 1988, p. v). It concluded that the nation "has lost sight of its public health goals and has allowed the system of public health activities to fall into disarray" and that the public health system was incapable of meeting its responsibilities (IOM, 1988).

The legal and constitutional framework in which public health activities are conducted contributes to the "disarray" and fractured system of public health identified by the IOM. A consequence of limited scope of federal government's authority in regulating health is that there is no central public health authority with nationwide reach; no entity or agency has comprehensive authority for the operation of the public health system. Instead, as the IOM observed, because public health regulations and services are implemented primarily at the state and local level, public health goals emerge within different political units and communities, each with their own health problems and concerns, political systems, resource availability, organizations, and values (IOM, 1988). Therefore, public health systems vary widely from community to community, with each prioritizing different problems and offering different responses and solutions to public health issues. While this characteristic may enhance local control, appropriateness, and flexibility of local agencies to meet the needs of a particular population, it also leads to fragmentation and uneven distribution in the type and quality of services provided (Baker et al., 2005). Further, with responsibility for health dispersed across federal, state, and local agencies and governments, coordination in the response to health problems or in pursuit of health goals is often frustrated by fragmented system organization. The division of authority has led to inconsistency, poor resource allocation, and lack of clarity about the agencies' respective responsibilities (Baker & Koplan, 2002). In light of this, the IOM concluded that "viewed from a national perspective, the national public health system is a scene of tremendous variety and disarray as different communities work out different solutions to public health problems" (IOM, 1988, p. 74).

The IOM did not conclude that the structure of the U.S. public health system was inherently flawed. Rather, it acknowledged that states have primary authority over public health matters, that local health departments provide the "front" line in the delivery of public health services, and that the federal government has the resources to facilitate improvement of the public health infrastructure. It emphasized that no community should be without the protections of a public health system, and concluded that this was possible only through the local components of an organized nationwide system of state-level agencies (IOM, 1988; Tilson & Berkowitz, 2006). Rather than propose a reorganization of the public health system, the IOM concentrated on the enterprise of public health, and identified three core functions that should be conducted by public health agencies at all levels of government: (a) assessment—activities concerning community diagnosis such as surveillance and epidemiology; (b) policy development—determination and prioritization of problems, goals, solutions, and resource allocation; and (c) assurance—guaranteeing that necessary public health services are provided. The IOM acknowledge that implementation of the core functions would vary from place to place. "The specific actions appropriate to strengthen public health will vary from area to area and must blend professional knowledge with community values" (IOM, 1988, p. 18).

10 Essential Services

In 1994, the DHHS convened a committee with representatives from all major public health constituencies, including the American Public Health Association (APHA), the Association of Schools of Public Health (ASPH), the ASTHO, the Environmental Council of the States (ECS), the NACCHO, the National Association of State Alcohol and Drug Abuse Directors, the National Association of State Mental Health Program Directors, the Public Health Foundation (PHF), and the divisions of DHHS constituting the U.S. Public Health Service. The Public Health Functions Steering Committee released a consensus statement titled, *Public Health in America*, which stated the vision, mission, purposes, and essential functions of public health in the United States (Public Health Functions Steering Committee, Office of Disease Prevention and Health Promotion, Office of Public Health and Science, U.S. Department of Health and Human Services, 1994). According to the statement, public health:

- Prevents epidemics and the spread of disease,
- Protects against environmental hazards,
- Prevents injuries,
- Promotes and encourages healthy behaviors,
- Responds to disasters and assists communities in recovery, and
- Assures the quality and accessibility of health services.

The committee also identified 10 essential services of public health, which have come to guide the practice of public health:

- Monitor health status to identify community health problems.
- Diagnose and investigate health problems and health hazards in the community.
- Inform, educate, and empower people about health issues.
- Mobilize community partnerships to identify and solve health problems.
- Develop policies and plans that support individual and community health efforts.
- Enforce laws and regulations that protect health and ensure safety.
- Link people to needed personal health services and ensure the provision of health care when otherwise unavailable.
- Ensure a competent public health and personal health care workforce.
- Evaluate effectiveness, accessibility, and quality of personal and population-based health services.
- Research for new insights and innovative solutions to health problems.

The list of 10 essential services translates the three core functions identified by the IOM into a more specific set of activities. These embody the protections and services that every citizen has the right to expect and every government has the obligation to assure. No matter what the unique features of any single community, the concept of the 10 essential services recognizes that every community needs a robust and reliable agency infrastructure" (Tilson & Berkowitz, 2006). The 10 essential services now provide the foundation for the nation's public health strategy, including the *Healthy People 2010* objectives, which will be discussed in Chapter 6, and the development of the National Public Health Performance Standards (CDC, 2007; DHHS, 2000).

FEDERAL PUBLIC HEALTH

Despite the constitutional restrictions on the federal government's role in regulating public health, it nevertheless plays a very large role in the U.S. public health system. The two powers constitutionally delegated to the federal government mentioned before—the power to tax and spend for the general welfare and the power to regulate interstate commerce—provide the basis for most federal activity in the public health arena. The federal government's key activities can generally be categorized as falling under at least one of four groups: (a) allocation and distribution of resources to public health actors; (b) information generation and distribution; (c) health care access assurance; and (d) regulation and enforcement. In many cases, an activity may be characterized as falling under more than one category.

The power to tax and spend is exactly what it sounds like: the federal government is authorized to collect and distribute funds to promote the welfare of the nation. "Spending" may be either the funding of projects and programs carried out by the government itself, financing contracts with external parties, or making direct contributions of fund (e.g., through grants). Most of the federal government's public health activities are based on its power to tax and spend. For example, pursuant to this power, the federal government conducts extensive health monitoring, surveillance, and epidemiological studies; it conducts and funds health and biomedical research; it surveys the nation's health status and health needs; it develops policies, guidelines, and standards for public health practice; it provides direct and indirect funding to state and local public health agencies, as well as private organizations such as community health centers; it supports public information and education campaigns on health-related matters; it conducts and funds public health education and research; it provides education and training to the public health workforce; and it funds or provides access to personal health services though such programs as community health centers, Medicaid, Medicare, State Children's Health Insurance Program (SCHIP), and health care for veterans. The taxing power is also used to encourage or discourage certain behaviors. For example, the federal government may encourage private business to provide health insurance to employees through tax credits, and it may discourage the consumption of tobacco products or alcohol through the imposition of excise or "sin" taxes.

The federal government's health-related regulatory authority is generally derived from the Commerce Clause—the constitutional provision permitting the federal government to regulate interstate commerce. Although generally more limited in scope than its activities financing public health research and services or providing access to health care, the federal government does impose and enforce regulations and laws in several public health areas affecting the country generally. For example, federal agencies enforce regulations concerning drug, food, and occupational safety, as well as environmental protection. The federal government's regulatory activities in each of these arenas are based in its authority under the Commerce Clause. If there were political will, this could be overcome and the federal control imposed. See clean air act case; same reasoning could be applied to communicable disease monitoring—disease affects business and does not respect political boundaries.

Department of Health and Human Services: Public Health Service[1]

The central, though not only, federal agency responsible for health and health care in the United States is the DHHS. Its mission is to act as "the United States government's principal agency for protecting the health of all Americans and [to] provid[e] essential human services, especially for those who are least able to help themselves" (DHHS, 2010a, para. 1). Through 11 operating divisions, DHHS administers more than 300 health-related pro-

---

[1] At the time this book was written, the DHHS was undergoing reorganization. Therefore, the organization of the offices, centers, and agencies within the DHHS is different. However, the essential services of each remain the same.

grams in a wide range of areas, including health and biomedical research, epidemiology and surveillance, disease prevention and immunization, food and drug safety, providing access to primary health care for certain populations, and bioterrorism response preparedness (DHHS, 2010b). DHHS directly employs the full time equivalent of approximately 70,000 people and in 2010 had a budget of $828 billion (DHHS, 2009).

Out of the 11 operating divisions within DHHS, 9 are components of the U.S. Public Health Service. There are three staff offices within the Office of the Secretary, which are also designated components of the U.S. Public Health Service and which operate to coordinate the agency's public health activities. These operating divisions and staff offices themselves each contain many subagencies and offices, administering hundreds of programs within DHHS. Table 3.1 lists the operating divisions and staff offices of the U.S. Public Health Service and their respective missions.

TABLE 3.1   Department of Health and Human Services, Operating Divisions and Staff Offices Constituting the U.S. Public Health Service

Agency for Healthcare Research and Quality (AHRQ)	Mission: to improve the quality, safety, efficiency, and effectiveness of health care for all Americans
Agency for Toxic Substances and Disease Registry[a] (ATSDR)	Mission: to serve the public through responsive public health actions to promote healthy and safe environments and prevent harmful exposures
Centers for Disease Control and Prevention (CDC)	Mission: collaborating to create the expertise, information, and tools that people and communities need to protect their health–through health promotion, prevention of disease, injury, and disability, and preparedness for new health threats
Food and Drug Administration (FDA)	Mission: (a) to protect the public health by ensuring the safety, efficacy, and security of human and veterinary drugs, biological products, medical devices, our nation's food supply, cosmetics, and products that emit radiation; (b) to advance the public health by helping to speed innovations that make medicines and foods more effective, safer, and more affordable; and helping the public get the accurate, science-based information they need to use medicines and foods to improve their health
Health Resources and Services Administration (HRSA)	Mission: to improve health and achieve health equity through access to quality services, a skilled health workforce and innovative programs

Indian Health Service (IHS)	*Mission:* to raise the physical, mental, social, and spiritual health of American Indians and Alaska Natives to the highest level
National Institutes of Health (NIH)	*Mission:* to seek fundamental knowledge about the nature and behavior of living systems and the application of that knowledge to enhance health, lengthen life, and reduce the burdens of illness and disability
Substance Abuse and Mental Health Services Administration (SAMHSA)	*Mission:* to reduce the impact of substance abuse and mental illness on America's communities
Staff Offices Within the Office of the Secretary	
Office of Public Health and Science (OPHS)	*Mission:* to promote, protect, and improve the nation's health by providing leadership to the nation on public health and science, coordinating public health and science activities across HHS, and communicating on these subjects to the American people
Office of the Assistant Secretary for Preparedness and Response (ASPR)	*Mission:* lead the nation in preventing, preparing for, and responding to the adverse health effects of public health emergencies and disasters
Office of Global Health Affairs (OGHA)	*Mission:* to promote the health of the world's population by advancing the secretary's and the Department of Health and Human Services' global strategies and partnerships, thus serving the health of the people of the United States

Note: DHHS, 2010a,b.
[a]Recently merged with the CDC's National Center for Environmental Health and is undergoing reorganization.

As Table 3.1 indicates, the scope of activities and services undertaken by the U.S. Public Health Service is vast, and indeed, many of the identified subagencies and offices have their own branches and divisions, each with its own mission and program responsibilities. A comprehensive discussion of the activities and programs of the U.S. Public Health Service agencies is far beyond what can be accomplished here. What follows should not, by any means, be considered an exhaustive description of the agencies discussed, but is rather intended to give an idea of some of the key programs and activities of the U.S. Public Health Service agencies, and how the federal government supports the 10 essential public health services.

Centers for Disease Control and Prevention[2]

Established in 1946 as the Communicable Disease Center, the Centers for Disease Control and Prevention is the preeminent epidemiological, surveillance, and disease prevention agency in the federal government. Among its key functions is to monitor and report on the nation's health, detect health problems and disease outbreaks, research and implement disease prevention strategies, develop and advocate sound public health policies, promote healthy behaviors, and provide public health leadership and training. The CDC is the nation's go-to agency for public health. It is the voice of public health for the nation. The CDC houses some of the best epidemiologists, biomedical, behavioral, and social scientists, prevention researchers, health policy analysts, and health economists in the world. Many know the CDC for its outstanding work related to infectious diseases. Its staff travels to sites worldwide when infectious disease outbreaks occur. The CDC publishes the essential *Morbidity and Mortality Weekly Report* (MMWR), which contains the latest information on reportable diseases, new hazards, and other emerging health conditions. The CDC has also been a leader in bioterrorism threats research and practice. The CDC has become actively involved in noninfectious disease prevention, as well as the area of chronic diseases and injury control. Employing the equivalent of nearly 10,000 full-time employees (DHHS, 2009), the CDC has been called "the nation's premier and largest public health organization" (Hartsaw, 2009, p. 141). The scope of its activities is too great to be presented here, but a few examples follow.

Infectious Diseases

At present, the CDC has three centers to prevent, control, and detect communicable diseases: the National Center for Immunization and Respiratory Diseases; National Center for Emerging and Zoonotic Infectious Diseases (NCEZD); and National Center for HIV/AIDS, Viral Hepatitis, STD, and TB Prevention.

---

[2] At the time of writing, many divisions of the CDC are undergoing a reorganization, which is not yet complete. For example, the National Center for Preparedness, Detection, and Control of Infectious Diseases and the National Center for Zoonotic, Vector-Borne, and Enteric Diseases are being realigned into a single center called The National Center for Emerging and Zoonotic Infectious Diseases. Where possible, we discuss the roles and activities of the new centers, even if integration of the divisions is not yet completed

The *National Center for Immunization and Respiratory Diseases*, through its Division of Bacterial Diseases provides bacterial disease outbreak response, diagnostic epidemiology, vaccine development, and control for respiratory and vaccine-preventable disease. The center's Immunization Services Division provides financial support for the purchase of vaccines and immunization programs, provides provider and public education, and conducts and finances vaccine evaluation and research. Among the key vaccine programs administered by the CDC are the congressionally mandated Vaccines for Children Program, as well as a discretionary vaccine program. Together, these programs constitute a nearly $4 billion immunization program (DHHS, 2009). Through the Vaccines for Children Program, recommended vaccines are provided at no cost to children 18 years of age or younger who are Medicaid eligible, uninsured, American Indians and Alaska Natives, or who receive their immunizations at federally qualified health centers and lack insurance coverage for vaccines. The program provides 43% of all childhood vaccines for children younger than 7 years and 26% of vaccines for 7- to 18-year-olds (DHHS, 2009). The CDC also provides approximately $560 million in discretionary funding to support state immunization infrastructure and operational costs as well as to underwrite the cost of many of the vaccines provided by state and local public health departments to individuals not otherwise eligible under the Vaccines for Children Program, including adults (DHHS, 2009).

The *NCEZD* works to detect, prevent, and control the spread of infectious diseases, focusing on zoonotic diseases (which account for 75% of recently emerging infectious diseases), diseases found in connection with refugee health, foodborne diseases, waterborne diseases, nosocomial (health care-associated) infections, and vectorborne diseases. Within the several divisions comprising the office, CDC conducts extensive disease epidemiology, laboratory programs, and basic and applied research relating to infectious disease; plans for and coordinates prevention and outbreak response; and through Division of Preparedness and Emerging Infections, supports the development of prevention and control capacity across the nation. NCEZD also administers the CDC's quarantine stations—the 20 sites located at major ports of entry and land-border crossing at which the CDC health officers decide whether ill persons or certain products can enter the United States to prevent the spread of infectious diseases.

The *National Center for HIV/AIDS, Viral Hepatitis, STD, and TB Prevention* is responsible for public health surveillance, prevention research, and programs to prevent and control human immunodeficiency virus (HIV) and acquired immune deficiency syndrome (AIDS), sexually transmitted diseases (STDs), viral hepatitis, and tuberculosis (TB). The center works in collaboration with governmental and nongovernmental partners at community, state, and national levels on research, surveillance, technical assistance, evaluation, and development of prevention programs.

Noninfectious Diseases and Injuries

Many units within the CDC focus on noninfectious diseases and injuries: Office of Noncommunicable Diseases, Injury and Environmental Health; National Center for Chronic Disease Prevention and Health Promotion; National Center for Environmental Health; Agency for Toxic Substances and Disease Registry (ATSDR), National Center for Injury Prevention and Control; National Institute for Occupational Safety and Health (NIOSH); and National Center on Birth Defects and Developmental Disabilities.

The *Office of Noncommunicable Diseases, Injury and Environmental Health* works to prevent and control chronic diseases. Focusing on many of the leading causes of morbidity and mortality such as cancer, diabetes, heart disease and stroke, nutrition/obesity, and tobacco use, the center provides funding and assistance to help state, tribal, and territorial health agencies to support data collection on disease risk factors, incidence, and death; to conduct research on disease risk and prevention strategies; to implement disease prevention programs; and to provide educational materials for health professionals, policymakers, and the public on issues pertaining to chronic disease prevention and control.

Among the programs administered by the *National Center for Chronic Disease Prevention and Health Promotion* is the Preventive Health and Health Services Block Grant program, which provides funds to state-level agencies to support both public health agency capacity development and chronic disease prevention programs. Grants made under the $100 million annual program are designed to be flexible, providing states funding to fill gaps in programs that address the leading causes of death and disability in a manner defined determined by the grantees based on the particular needs of the population served. The funds are frequently used to support clinical services, preventative screening, public education, workforce development, surveillance, and chronic disease prevention programs.

The *National Center for Environmental Health* works to prevent illness, disability, and death resulting from human interaction with environmental toxins. The center conducts surveillance and applied research, supports educational campaigns, develops standards and guidelines, and offers training to state and local health agencies in environmental health prevention and response. It works in conjunction with the *ATSDR*, a congressionally mandated agency charged with conducting public health assessments of waste sites, conducting health surveillance and registries related to toxic substances, and providing information, education, and training concerning hazardous substances.

The *National Center for Injury Prevention and Control* works to prevent injuries and violence, and reduce their consequences. The center conducts injury and violent death surveillance, and supports research and injury prevention programs in such areas as domestic violence. The center also funds extramural research on injury prevention, care, and rehabilitation, and supports Injury Control Research Centers at several academic institutions across the country.

The *NIOSH*, created in conjunction with the U.S. Department of Labor's Occupational Safety and Health Administration (OSHA). Whereas OSHA has the responsibility of developing and enforcing workplace safety and health regulations, NIOSH was formed to provide the research in the field of occupational safety and health necessary to do so effectively. NIOSH conducts research, develops guidance and recommendations on workplace safety, disseminates information, and upon request, conducts workplace health hazard evaluations. In addition to its own research, NIOSH sponsors research and training through extramural programs and enters cooperative agreements with state health departments, academia, unions, and NGOs to participate in collaborative surveillance and research projects.

The *National Center on Birth Defects and Developmental Disabilities* conducts research and supports extramural research designed to identify the causes of birth defects and developmental disabilities and to promote the well-being of persons with disabilities. The center also funds prevention and education programs.

National Center for Health Statistics

The National Center for Health Statistics (NCHS) is the premier organization for the collection, processing, analysis, and dissemination of health data for the nation. The NCHS collects "data from birth and death records, medical records, interview surveys, and through direct physical exams and laboratory testing" (NCHS, 2010a, para. 3). Major regular surveys and data collection systems of the NCHS, from which information is drawn about the nation's health and the determinants of health include the following (NCHS, 2010b):

- National Health and Nutrition Examination Survey (NHANES)
  - Continuous NHANES
  - NHANES III
  - NHANES II
  - NHANES I
  - NHANES Epidemiologic Follow-Up Study (NHEFS)
  - Hispanic HANES
  - National Health Examination Survey (NHES)
- National Health Care Surveys (NHCS)
  - National Ambulatory Medical Care Survey (NAMCS)
  - National Hospital Ambulatory Medical Care Survey (NHAMCS)
  - National Hospital Discharge Survey (NHDS)
  - National Survey of Ambulatory Surgery (NSAS)
  - National Home and Hospice Care Survey (NHHCS)
  - National Home Health Aide Survey (NHHAS)
  - National Nursing Home Survey (NNHS)
  - National Nursing Assistant Survey (NNAS)
  - National Survey of Residential Care Facilities (NSRCF)
- National Health Interview Survey (NHIS)
  - National Health Interview Survey on Disability (NHIS-D)
  - Joint Canada/United States Survey of Health (JCUSH)
- National Immunization Survey (NIS)
- National Survey of Family Growth (NSFG)
- National Vital Statistics System (NVSS)
  - Birth Data
  - Mortality Data
  - Fetal Death Data
  - Linked Births/Infant Deaths
  - National Mortality Followback Survey
  - National Maternal and Infant Health Survey
- The Longitudinal Studies of Aging (LSOA)
- State and Local Area Integrated Telephone Survey (SLAITS)

Data from the NCHS surveys and systems are available to the public through the NCHS Web site (http://www.cdc.gov/nchs/) as public-use files. The NCHS also produces innumerable standardized reports based on these data. The NCHS data are essential for developing, implementing, and evaluating public health policy in the United States. They allow:

- Documentation of population and subpopulation health status;
- Identification of health and health care disparities by race or ethnicity, socioeconomic status, region, and other population characteristics;
- Description of health care system experiences;
- Monitoring health status and health care delivery trends;
- Identification of health problems;
- Support of biomedical and health services research;
- Provision of information for policy; and
- Evaluation of health policies and programs impact (NCHS, 2010a).

Other Centers for Disease Control and Prevention Offices and Centers

Other offices and centers include the Office of Surveillance, Epidemiology, and Laboratory Services; Office of Public Health Preparedness and Response; Office for State, Tribal, Local and Territorial Support; and Center for Global Health. The CDC's *Office for State, Tribal, Local and Territorial Support* aims to improve the capacity and performance of the public health system at all levels of organization by providing guidance on activities related to state, tribal and local, and public health agencies. The office provides technical assistance and direct funding to state and local agencies to support the delivery of public health services and programs in accordance with CDC guidelines and standards in areas such as health promotion and disease prevention, public health policy, technology and communications infrastructure, and workforce development.[3]

Through its *Center for Global Health*, CDC works with international partners to prevent and control infectious and chronic diseases and to build sustainable global public health capacity through the development of epidemiological and laboratory resources and the international public health workforce. Activities of the *Center for Global Health* include programs in global disease detection through which the CDC works with international public health actors such as ministries of health and the World Health Organization to develop capacity for the rapid detection, identification, and containment of infectious diseases and bioterrorist threats internationally.

---

[3]http://www.cdc.gov/ostlts/

The Center for Global Health also supports programs in AIDS prevention and treatment, and the prevention and control or eradication of polio, measles, influenza, and malaria. CDC staff work in more than 50 countries in support of the global health mission.

Agency for Healthcare Research and Quality

The Agency for Healthcare Research and Quality (AHRQ) is the lead federal agency charged with improving the quality, safety, efficiency, and effectiveness of health care for all Americans. It does not make policy, but rather, with a budget of approximately $372 million and a staff of 300,[4] AHRQ "conducts and sponsors health services research to inform decision making and improve clinical care and the organization and financing of health care" (DHHS, 2010c). AHRQ's research, which is both conducted internally and through grants and contracts to universities, health care systems, hospitals, and physician practices, focuses on a set of broad issues relating to both clinical services and the system in which those services are provided, including comparative effectiveness, patient safety, health information technology, prevention and care management for chronic conditions, and value research.

Among the programs supported by AHRQ are 12 Evidence-Based Practice Centers, established to review and synthesize available evidence on various health care topics and to assess and describe the quality of the evidence. AHRQ also supports 14 Centers for Education and Research on Therapeutics charged with developing and disseminating information concerning products that may be used to prevent or treat disease. The purpose of the centers is to enable appropriate use of available drugs and products to facilitate safe and effective use and treatment while reducing cost. AHRQ also administers the Health Care Cost and Utilization Program, through which it collects and distributes statistical data related to hospital inpatient care from across the nation.

Health Resources and Services Administration

The activities of the Health Resources and Services Administration (HRSA) are principally to further the essential services related to workforce development and ensuring access to health care services. Comprising 6 bureaus and 13 offices and with a staff more than 1,600, HRSA is the primary federal

---

[4] http://www.ahrq.gov/about/ataglance.htm

agency for improving access to health care services for people who are un-insured, isolated, or particularly vulnerable. HRSA provides leadership and financial support to health care providers in every state and U.S. territory.[5] Primarily a grant-giving and oversight agency, HRSA distributes the over-whelming majority of its budget to community-based organizations, colleges and universities, hospitals, local and state governments, associations, and foundations.

HRSA's Bureau of Clinician Recruitment and Service provides scholar-ship and educational loan repayment opportunities in exchange for clini-cians' agreement to serve in communities with critical shortages of health care providers. The Bureau of Health Professions similarly supports work-force development by making grants to health professions training pro-grams and funding scholarships and loan repayment programs for health professionals.

HRSA's HIV/AIDS Bureau administers the Ryan White HIV/AIDS Program, which provides funding to grantees for HIV/AIDS outreach and AIDS Drug Assistance Programs (ADAPs). The program is designed to help those who do not have sufficient health care coverage or financial resources to cope with HIV and AIDS. The Maternal and Child Health Bureau ad-ministers the Maternal and Child Health Block Grant to states. The grants are designed to expand access to comprehensive prenatal and postnatal care for women, support health assessments, diagnostics, and treatment for children, and expand access to immunization and other preventive care for children.

HRSA's Bureau of Primary Health Care provides funding for nonprofit, community-run health centers delivering comprehensive primary and pre-ventative health care for people who otherwise lack access to health care. Populations served by these centers include people with low incomes, the uninsured, those with limited English proficiency, migrant and seasonal farm workers, individuals and families who are homeless, and those living in public housing. Health centers provide care on a sliding fee scale and see patients without regard for their ability to pay. There are approximately 1,200 community health organizations, delivering health care services at 8,000 sites. The centers serve approximately 20 million people, including nearly 1 million migrant farm workers and 1 million homeless persons. There were approximately 67 million patient visits to federally funded health centers in 2008 (HRSA, 2010).

---

[5]http://www.hrsa.gov/about/index.html

Food and Drug Administration

The Food and Drug Administration (FDA), with approximately 11,500 employees, is the agency charged with regulating drugs and most food products in the United States. Over-the-counter and prescription drugs, including generic drugs, are regulated by FDA's Center for Drug Evaluation and Research. The FDA evaluates drug safety and efficacy and ensures that the labeling and marketing of approved drugs is accurate. Vaccines, blood, and biologics are regulated by FDA's Center for Biologics Evaluation and Research. The Center for Food Safety and Applied Nutrition works to ensure that the food supply is safe, sanitary, and honestly labeled. The Center for Tobacco Products was established to oversee the regulation of the marketing and promotion of tobacco products and set performance standards for tobacco products to protect the public health. The FDA also operates the National Center for Toxicological Research, which conducts research aimed at the evaluation of biological effects of potentially toxic chemicals or microorganisms and to understand toxicological processes so as to inform the FDA's regulatory decisions.

National Institutes of Health

The National Institutes of Health (NIH) is the primary federal agency conducting and supporting biomedical research. Composed of 27 Institutes and Centers, the NIH conducts and funds research into the causes, treatment, cure, and prevention of a broad range of disease. The vast majority of NIH's budget goes to support extramural research at universities and other research institutions. Included in its portfolio is a substantial body of disease prevention research. Research on disease prevention is an important part of the NIH mission. The Institutes and Centers have a broad portfolio of prevention research and training, as well as programs to disseminate the findings to scientists, health professionals, and the public. Ultimately, knowledge gained from NIH-supported prevention research enables the application of sound science in clinical practice, health policy, and community health programs, thereby improving the health of the public.

Indian Health Service

The Indian Health Service (IHS) is responsible for providing federal health services to American Indians and Alaska Natives. The IHS provides a comprehensive health service delivery system for approximately 1.9 million American Indians and Alaskan Natives who belong to 564 federally recognized tribes in 35 states. It is the principal federal health care provider and health advocate for native people. The IHS operates or finances 45 hospitals, nearly 300 health centers, and numerous other community clinics, health stations, and school health centers.

In addition to providing direct health care services, the IHS also undertakes broader health promotion activities. For example, the Office of Environmental Health and Engineering promotes the development of safe water and waste treatment programs. The IHS has also launched a Health Promotion and Disease Prevention (HP/DP) Initiative that aims to develop and implement effective health promotion and chronic disease prevention programs, particularly in areas of concern for the native population including increasing incidence of chronic diseases related to lifestyle issues such as obesity, physical inactivity, poor diet, substance abuse, and injuries.

Substance Abuse and Mental Health Services Administration

The Substance Abuse and Mental Health Services Administration (SAMHSA) works to improve the quality and availability of substance abuse prevention, addiction treatment, and mental health services. SAMHSA provides funding through block grants to state and local governments to support substance abuse and mental health services, including treatment for serious substance abuse problems or mental health problems; supports education programs for the general public and health care providers; improves substance abuse prevention and treatment services through the identification and dissemination of best practices; and conducts surveillance and monitoring of the prevalence and incidence of substance abuse.

Other Department of Health and Human Services Divisions

Although not designated components of the U.S. Public Health Service, other divisions of DHHS also perform important public health services. For example, the *Administration on Aging* supports programs related to the long-term care of the elderly, including nutrition programs, as well as health and prevention programs related to long-term chronic disease and disability. Most notable, however, are DHHS activities in the area of ensuring access to health services. In particular, the *Centers for Medicare & Medicaid Services* (CMS) administer the largest insurance programs in the country, with a combined budget of approximately $760 billion annually. Medicare provides publicly financed health insurance for more than 44.6

million elderly and disabled Americans, and Medicaid, a program administered jointly by the federal government and the states, provides publicly financed health coverage for approximately 50 million low-income earner persons and nursing home coverage for low-income earner elderly adults. CMS also administers the SCHIP that covers more than 4.4 million children. Together, the Medicare and Medicaid programs provide health care access to nearly one third of the U.S. population. Although primarily considered a health care insurance program for low-income earner people, Medicaid-reimbursed services may also include such public health activities as Early and Periodic Screening, Diagnostic, and Treatment (EPSDT) services for children, family planning services, cancer screening, school health services, and adult immunizations. Further, Medicaid payments also support public health providers such as health centers, public hospitals, community mental health providers, and STD clinics, which are dependent on Medicaid revenues to sustain their operations (Perlino, 2006).

Other Federal Agencies

Federal agencies other than those in DHHS have important public health roles. These include the U.S. Department of Agriculture (USDA), Environmental Protection Agency, U.S. Department of Labor, and the VA and the Department of Defense.

U.S. Department of Agriculture

The USDA plays a vital regulatory role in the public health system through its Food Safety and Inspection Service, the public health agency responsible for the safety and labeling of the commercial supply of meat, poultry, and egg products. The USDA also plays a role in directly ensuring health through its Food and Nutrition Service, which oversees funding of food assistance programs such as the Supplemental Nutrition Assistance Program (formerly the Food Stamp Program), which subsidizes food purchases for 28 million people each month; the National School Lunch Program, which provides subsidies to schools for meals in exchange for serving lunches to students who meet federal nutritional requirements and offering free or reduced price lunches to eligible children; and the Women Infants and Children Program (WIC), which provides federal grants to states for supplemental foods, health care referrals, and nutrition education for low-income earner pregnant, breastfeeding, and nonbreastfeeding postpartum women and to infants and children up to age 5 who are found to be at nutritional risk.

Environmental Protection Agency

The Environmental Protection Agency regulates the release of pollutants in the air, land, and water and conducts or provides grants for environmental remediation where necessary. Among the laws administered by the EPA are the Clean Air Act, the Clean Water Act, the Comprehensive Environmental Response, Compensation and Liability Act, and the Toxic Substances Control Act. Nearly half of EPA's budget is expended through grants to states, nonprofits, educational institutions, and others for various projects, from scientific studies to site cleanups.

U.S. Department of Labor

The U.S. Department of Labor, through the OSHA, regulates the health and safety of workplaces, either directly or through approval of state occupational safety programs that exceed federal requirements. OSHA regulations are based on NIOSH research and regulate matters ranging from the permissible exposures limits for hazardous substances in the workplace to the use of portable power tools.

Department of Veterans Affairs and Department of Defense

The Department of Veterans Affairs (VA) and the Department of Defense provide access to health care services to veterans and active military personnel. The VA operates the nation's largest integrated health care system, with a network of 153 medical centers, more than 800 community-based outpatient clinics, 135 nursing homes, 46 residential rehabilitation treatment programs, and 207 readjustment counseling centers. In 2009, it provided care to nearly 5.5 million veterans and more than 54 million outpatient visits (U.S. Department of Veterans Affairs, 2010).

STATE PUBLIC HEALTH

As described earlier, the primary legal authority for public health in the United States rests with the states. Although the federal government undertakes extensive public health activities, as we have seen, those programs are generally categorized under resource allocation and distribution, information generation and distribution, health care access assurance, and, to a more limited extent, regulation and enforcement in matters affecting the country broadly (e.g., drug and food safety). The states generally have responsibility, at least at first, for implementing public health programs and delivering public health services. So while the federal government has, for example, established the National Electronic Disease Surveillance System whereby state and local health agencies may report incidences of reportable diseases, the decision whether or to what degree to participate in the system is left to the states, individually. The ASTHO—citing considerable variation among agencies—finds the public health system "comprehensive, yet inconsistent" (ASTHO, 2009, p. 8).

Organization and Governance

There is at least one state-level government authority with primary responsibility for public health in every state, and in state governments alone, there are more than 100,000 workers in the area of public health (ASTHO, 2008). State health departments are structured and organized in a multitude of ways, are located in different parts of state government, and differ in the extent and nature of the authority granted to them. In general, state public health departments are organized in one of three ways. Stand-alone agencies are independent from other agencies. They are mixed-function agencies (sometimes referred to as "super agencies") that are independent but also carry out activities other than core public health activities, such as health insurance regulation or Medicaid administration. Most state health departments (55%) are freestanding, independent agencies of these sorts.

Other state health departments are part of a larger "umbrella" agency of state government, such as a state department of health and human services, which oversees several departments. In states where the health department falls within an umbrella agency, other health services are often provided by other departments of the agency, including administration of the state Medicaid program, provision of long-term care services, substance abuse treatment and prevention or other behavioral health services, and environmental protection (ASTHO, 2009). The California Department of Public Health is one example of a public health department located within an umbrella agency: the California Health and Human Services Agency (CHHSA). CHHSA oversees 12 departments other than Public Health, including the departments of Aging, Alcohol and Drug Programs, Health Care Services (Medicaid and other public insurance administration), Mental Health, and Social Services.

State public health agencies also vary in the authorities granted to them. Most state health departments (70%) are authorized to declare health emergencies and to collect key health data. Less than one half of state health departments, however, have the authority to adopt public health laws and regulations. Health departments have even less authority over budgetary and leadership issues. Overall funding and administrative decisions generally rest with the legislature or executive branch of state government. For example, less than 30% of state health agencies have budget authority, and almost none may select the agency head, establish taxes in support of public health, or place tax and levy measures on the ballot; those powers being reserved for the governor or legislature (ASTHO, 2009).

Twenty-six states have boards or councils of health, which variously promulgate rules and advise elected officials on policy. A minority of state boards of health formulate public health policies, legislative agendas, or public health budgets for the state (Beitsch, Brooks, Grigg, & Menachemi, 2006). In 12% of states, the state board of health has primary responsibility for public health, whereas the state health official has primary responsibility in 64% of states (ASTHO, 2009). Boards of health, typically comprised of citizens, consumers, members of the business community, and public health professionals, play a decreasingly important role in state public health activities (Beitsch et al., 2006).

The relationship between state health departments and local departments also exhibits considerable variation. The survey data on the governance and organizational relationship are not entirely consistent, but generally, between 12% and 20% of states are best characterized as having state health department control over local health departments; between 37% and 57% of local health departments are decentralized, operating independently (though often in collaboration with) state health agencies; and between 26% and 35% of states have a mix, with some local health agencies acting independently and some under the direction of the state agency (ASTHO, 2009; NACCHO, 2009).

The overwhelming majority of state health agencies report partnering with NGOs on various programs and activities. Most frequently, state agencies partner with universities and schools, community organizations, hospitals and other health care providers, insurers, and community health centers. More than half of state agencies also report partnering with businesses, the media, and environmental and conservation organizations.

Services and Activities

State public health departments engage in wide range of public health activities. The top three activities reported by state health agencies were wellness and disease prevention programs, emergency preparedness, and epidemiology/ surveillance/monitoring. Notably, however, there is wide variety. No more than 40% identified disease prevention as a top three priority, and fewer than 30% identified emergency preparedness or epidemiology/surveillance as being one of their top three activities. Other "top three activities" included wellness, health promotion, health communication, improving performance, specific prevention programs (cancer control, immunizations, family and newborn screening, infant mortality reduction, as well as prevention programs for tobacco use, injury, and chronic diseases, most notably obesity and type 2 diabetes). Regulation, health insurance and health care, planning and policy, addressing health disparities, leadership development, adoption of National Public Health Performance Standards, implementation of the Public Health Improvement Project, workforce development, coordination with partners in the public health system, support for local public health agencies, and data driven management were also listed. The following is information about some of the major groupings of public health services and activities performed by states: surveillance and epidemiology, environmental health, maternal and child health, emergency preparedness, regulation, inspection, and licensing, and personal health care.

Surveillance and Epidemiology

Every state public health department conducts some level of public health surveillance, monitoring, and epidemiological activities in their state. All state public health departments monitor communicable and infectious diseases to some degree, and more than 90% of departments also monitor vital statistics, cancer incidence, perinatal events or risk factors, behavioral risk factors, chronic diseases, environmental health, and injury. The departments often engage in surveillance activities in connection with local public health authorities as well as the CDC.

Environmental Health

The overwhelming majority of state health agencies (80%–95%) oversee environmental health epidemiology and food safety education. Less frequently, but in most instances, the state health agency is involved in toxicology, as well as radiation, radon, poison, vector control, indoor air quality, and water supply safety.

Maternal and Child Health

More than 90% of states offer services to children with special health care needs, and most states also administer the Women, Infants, and Children (WIC) nutrition program and provide family planning and prenatal care services. Fewer than half of all state health departments provide non-WIC maternal and child nutrition services, well-child services, early periodic screening, diagnosis and treatment programs, comprehensive health clinics through schools, primary care for children, daycare, or child nutrition programs. Only about 28% provide obstetrical care.

Emergency Preparedness

All state health agencies have some responsibility to prepare for disaster response and emergencies. All state health departments have responsibility for responding to communicable disease outbreaks, nearly all have responsibilities for responding to bioterrorism events, and almost 90% have responsibilities for responding to chemical, nuclear, and natural disasters.

Regulation, Inspection, and Licensing

Most state health agencies have some involvement (along with other agencies at the federal, state, and/or local level) in the regulation, inspection, and licensing of food processing businesses (78%), prisons (73%), waste disposal businesses (72%), hospice care (71%), laboratories (68%), food service establishments (64%), local public health agencies (65%), and hospitals (56%). Most state public health departments, however, do not license health professionals. This is typically a function of another agency or department of state government. Fewer than 25% of state health agencies directly license nurses, physicians, physician assistants or dentists. Vital and health statistics may start at the state or local government level. Marriage, births, and deaths are state or local functions. Notification of reportable diseases starts at local level and is sent to the state.

Personal Health Care

With the exception of HIV/AIDS and STDs, state health agencies generally do not provide treatment for communicable and chronic disease. Fewer than 50% provide any treatment for breast or cervical cancer, and fewer than 30% provide any treatment of colon cancer, diabetes, elevated blood lead, or asthma. Fewer than 15% provide any treatment for high blood pressure, coronary heart disease, or any other cancers. However, 12 states, run and operate TB hospitals. Most state health agencies provide or regulate at least some clinical services in oral health, emergency medical services, minority health, and rural health. A minority provide services for victims of sexual assault and violence, substance abuse prevention, or pharmacy services.

Priorities

More than 40% of state health agency officials listed in their top five priorities: (a) developing effective health policy, (b) assuring a local public health presence throughout the state, (c) assuring preparedness for a health emergency, (d) monitoring the health of the state's population, and (e) early detection/population protection measures.

State governments have the authority and responsibility to protect the welfare of the population within their borders. As stated earlier, some states carry out the essential functions, whereas others delegate these services and duties. States take responsibilities for high-level laboratories, data collection, assessments, and policies. Many states issue certification and licensing for personnel and facilities and are responsible for enforcing disciplinary actions because of wrongful actions by health providers. Since Medicaid is a state–federal program, usually the state department plays an important role in setting policies as well as, in many cases, providing assurance and assessment; sometimes a small percentage may be delegated to the county level. The state may have counties carry out the eligibility determination.

Other issues related to the organization of public health services at the state level concern the locus of responsibility. Is there a separate agency for environment and environmental health? Is public health responsible for mental health and substance abuse, or is there a separate agency? This would also be the case for aging and child health. If there are separate agencies, do they work and coordinate together in a positive way? These issues are answered differently in different states and have consequences for the coordination and provision of public health services.

Relationship to 10 Essential Health Services

Surveys of state public health agencies indicate that, in general, most states perform public health activities falling within each of the 10 essential services, although it is difficult to evaluate this assessment because public health services and activities are not organized by the essential services.

Most services are specific to a health problem, population, and/or behavior. HIV/AIDS, STDs, foodborne diseases, waterborne diseases, maternal and child health, emergency preparedness, injuries, childhood immunizations, smoking, obesity, and nutrition are common organizational groupings of public health services and activities. In each case, the 10 essential services may (or may not be) be relevant or provided.

For example, it is not clear whether HIV/AIDS programs are assessed (or should be assessed) on whether they offer all 10 essential services for the population they serve: monitor, diagnose and investigate health problems related to HIV/AIDS in the community; inform, educate, and empower people with HIV/AIDS; mobilize community partnerships to solve their problems; develop policies and plans to support HIV/AIDS patients' health efforts; enforce laws and regulations to protect people with AIDS/HIV; link people with HIV/AIDS to needed personal health services if otherwise unavailable; ensure a competent workforce to meet AID/HIS patients' needs; evaluate services for people with HIV/AIDS; and research innovative solutions to their health problems. Further, it would be difficult to determine if all essential services were provided to people with HIV/AIDS because some essential services might be within the scope of the HIV/AIDS program and others might be within the responsibility of a crosscutting unit such as communications or epidemiology.

Also, it is difficult to compare across states on the essential services, because even though two states may conduct performance evaluations, the scope and depth of the evaluations undertaken may vary significantly, and the states may prioritize performance evaluation very differently. Further, there is little data showing whether the form of essential service provided was tailored to the particular needs of the population, or whether, for example, it was performed in response to a federal categorical grant without a particular need in the community.

LOCAL PUBLIC HEALTH

The implementation and delivery of many, if not most, public health services occur at the local level—usually city, county, or region. Local health departments are on the front line of control of communicable diseases and noncommunicable hazardous exposures, as well as informing and educating communities about public health issues. However, local public health organizations collaborate with state and federal public health agencies and depend on their resources—data, skilled personnel, funds, and so forth—a great deal. In most states, the state and local public health agencies form a very connected system. The state may not provide direct services but offers a higher level of technical expertise at the research and policy level, which the local health department carries out.

There are enormous variations between local health departments, as we will discuss. It is almost true that if you have seen one local health department, you have seen one local health department. They differ between states and, within states, on organization, governance, services offered, and implementation strategies. Not surprisingly, a major factor driving variation is the size of the population served. There are approximately 2,800 total local health departments in the United States (NACCHO, 2009). The majority—64%—of local health departments serves jurisdictions with 50,000 or fewer people, and 43% of local health departments serve jurisdictions with fewer than 25,000 people. Although constituting a sizable majority of departments, the persons served in these jurisdictions constitute only 12% of the national population (NACCHO, 2009). Jurisdictions of 50,000–499,999 persons are served by 31% of local health departments and comprise 41% of the population. Local health departments serving large urban centers—departments in jurisdictions with 500,000 or more people—constitute only 5% of nationwide local health departments yet serve 46% of the United States population (NACCHO, 2009).

Organization and Governance

Nearly every state's population is served by local health departments (regional, county, municipal). The only exceptions are Hawaii and Rhode Island, which do not have any local or regional health agencies. In those states, the state health departments operate on behalf of local public health, and there are no administrative or service units with responsibility for the health of a substate jurisdiction (NACCHO, 2009).

The political units served and jurisdictional boundaries of local health departments vary throughout the country. At the county level, 60% of local health departments operate, 18% operate at the city, town, or township level, and 11% serve combined county–city jurisdictions. The jurisdictions of 11% of local departments do not conform to discrete substate political units but are organized to serve a multicounty, regional, or other local district area (NACCHO, 2009). In some instances, it may be that city or township health departments operate within counties that are also served by county health departments (IOM, 2003).

Local health departments also vary in their governance. In 29 states, the local health departments are primarily governed by local authorities—local boards of health or officials of a county or city. The local departments in 6 states—Arkansas, Delaware, Florida, Mississippi, South Carolina, and Vermont—are governed by state-level authorities. In 13 states, some local health departments are governed primarily at the local level, whereas others are governed by state authorities (NACCHO, 2009).

The majority—80%—of local health departments have associated local boards of health. Local boards of health are associated with a local health department less frequently where a department serves a large population; whereas, 87% of local health departments, which serve populations of less than 10,000, have an associated local board of health, only 38% departments serving more than 1 million persons have local boards (NACCHO, 2009).

In 15 states, all local health departments have an associated local board of health. In 16 states, more than half of all local health departments are associated with a local board of health, and in 12 states, fewer than half of the departments have an associated board. In 5 states—Delaware, Louisiana, Mississippi, New Mexico, and South Carolina—there are no local boards of health. Most local boards of health have the authority to adopt public health regulations (73%), set and impose fees for services (68%), approve the budget for the local health department (59%), and hire or fire the head of the department head (56%). Some local boards also request public health levies (32%) and have the authority to impose taxes to support public health activities (17%). Local health board members may be elected, appointed, or sit on the board by designation in their capacity as some other elected or appointed official. Some local boards of health are comprised of members selected in various ways, but 66% of boards report that at least some members are appointed, whereas only 14% report members directly elected to the board (NACCHO, 2009).

Workforce

The estimated number of local health department workers nationwide is 155,000. The median number of full-time employees in a U.S. local health department is 15, ranging from a median of 3 for departments serving a population of fewer than 10,000 people to a median of 584 full-time employees for departments serving more than a million people. The median number of local public health department workers per 100,000 persons in the population served is 48 (NACCHO, 2009, 2010).

Most local health department heads are full-time employees (86%). The highest educational level for heads of local public health departments was master's degree (39%), followed by bachelor's degree (29%), doctoral degree (18%), and associates degree (7%). The educational level of department heads varies considerably by the size of the population served, with 57% of department executives serving populations greater than 500,000 holding a doctoral degree. Only 11% of executives of departments serving fewer than 25,000 people hold doctoral degrees, with 60% holding an associate's or bachelor's degree as the highest degree (NACCHO, 2009, 2010).

The composition of the public health workforce, overall, is seen in Figure 3.1. The largest portion of the workforce is uncategorized (26%), the second larger portion is the clerical staff (23%), followed by nurses (21%).

The ability to use information technology is increasingly important to local public health departments. From 2005–2008, the number of information specialists employed in local health departments increased 13.3% and public information specialists increased 9.4%. The number of health educators employed in local health departments decreased by 20%, the number of epidemiologists decreased by 10.9%, the number of registered nurses decreased 9.6%, and the number of physicians decreased 6.2% (NACCHO, 2010).

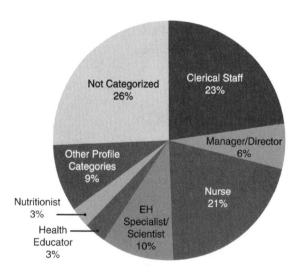

n ranged from 1,794 to 2,205 based on occupation
Note: Due to rounding, percentages do not add to 100.

FIGURE 3.1   Percentage Distribution of Occupations in the LHD Workforce

The composition of each local health department's workforce varies by size of the population served (see Table 3.2). The smallest departments often consist only of a director, secretary, and nurse. Next to be added are typically a sanitarian, health educator, and nutritionist. Nearly all of the largest departments have physicians, behavioral and environmental health scientists, epidemiologists, and information specialists, whereas these positions are rare in departments serving fewer than 100,000 people (NACCHO, 2009).

Services and Activities

As with the other characteristics examined, there is wide variation in the activities and services offered by local health departments. The activities and

TABLE 3.2   Percentage of Local Health Departments With Employees in Selected Occupations by Size of Population Served, 2008

	All Depts.	< 10,000	10,000–24,999	25,000–49,999	50,000–99,999	100,000–249,999	250,000–499,999	500,000–999,999	1,000,000+
Clerical staff	95%	85%	95%	97%	97%	100%	100%	100%	100%
Nurse	94%	82%	94%	96%	97%	98%	100%	97%	100%
Manager/director	91%	79%	89%	94%	96%	97%	100%	97%	100%
Environmental health specialist (sanitarian)	80%	54%	78%	86%	90%	92%	93%	88%	88%
Emergency preparedness coordinator	57%	38%	43%	52%	66%	77%	94%	96%	100%
Health educator	56%	25%	40%	57%	70%	78%	87%	96%	97%
Nutritionist	51%	23%	35%	50%	64%	76%	85%	85%	88%
Physician	42%	15%	24%	41%	52%	69%	79%	85%	94%
Behavioral Health professional	33%	6%	22%	26%	47%	49%	68%	80%	71%
Other environmental health scientist	27%	7%	17%	24%	32%	41%	65%	69%	70%
Information systems specialist	24%	4%	9%	16%	24%	49%	69%	86%	88%
Epidemiologist	23%	4%	7%	11%	19%	50%	78%	91%	100%

services most frequently offered directly by local health departments are the provision of adult immunizations (88% of departments), communicable and infectious disease surveillance (88% of departments), provision of child immunizations (86% of departments), TB screening (81% of departments), inspection of food service establishments (77% of departments), environmental health surveillance (75% of departments), food safety education (74% of departments), TB treatment (72% of departments), tobacco use prevention (70% of departments), and school and daycare inspection (68% of departments). The availability of the services varies with the size of the population served. For example, 79% of departments serving populations smaller than 25,000 people offer child immunization services, while 93% of departments serving more than 500,000 people do so. To state that the local health department does not provide a service either directly or through contract does not necessarily indicate that those services are not publicly available within a jurisdiction. In some cases, another local government agency, a state agency, or an NGO may provide the service. Following is a brief description of some of the common public health services and programs at the local level (NACCHO, 2009, 2010).

Surveillance and Epidemiology

Of all the local health departments studied, 88% perform surveillance and epidemiology with respect to communicable and infectious diseases, 75% perform surveillance in environmental health, and 61% do so in maternal and child health. A minority of departments conduct syndromic surveillance (40%), chronic disease surveillance (39%), surveillance of behavioral risk factors (33%), and injury surveillance (33%). Departments serving large populations are substantially more likely to perform epidemiology and surveillance.

Of all the local health departments studied, 81% provide screening for TB, and 68% do so for high blood pressure, 62% for blood lead, 60% for sexually transmitted diseases, 59% for HIV and AIDS, 45% for diabetes, 42% for cancer, and 35% for cardiovascular disease. For all of these conditions with exception of high blood pressure, the larger the population served by the local health department, the more likely the department is to offer screening. For example, less than half of departments serving fewer than 25,000 people offer screening for HIV/AIDS or STDs, whereas nearly 90% of departments serving more than 500,000 people do. Similarly, TB screening is available from the local health department in 72% of jurisdictions with fewer than 25,000 people but available in more than 90% of jurisdictions with populations of 100,000 or more.

Primary Prevention

Of all the local health departments studied, 70% engaged in primary prevention services concerning tobacco use, and 68% provided nutrition services. Approximately half of all departments offer prevention programs in the areas of chronic disease, exercise and physical activity, and unintended pregnancy. Other prevention services are less common, with injury prevention services available through 39% of departments, substance abuse prevention in 24%, violence prevention in 22%, and mental illness prevention services available in just 12%. Departments serving large populations are significantly more likely to offer prevention services than departments serving small populations. Notably, the four preventive services for which most departments do not offer are still reported to be available in a sizable majority of jurisdictions but are frequently provided by other government agencies or NGOs.

Maternal and Child Health

Of all the departments studied, 63% provide maternal and child health home visits, 62% provide WIC services, 54% provide family planning services, 44% provide services in connection with the Early Periodic Screening, Detection, and Treatment program (the child health component of Medicaid), 41% provide a Well-Child Clinic, 33% offer prenatal care, and 10% offer obstetrical care. Large public health departments are significantly more likely to offer these services than departments serving small populations.

Emergency Preparedness

Emergency preparedness has become a significant local health department effort as a result of 9/11 and the subsequent shift in funds and priority to this area at the federal level. Of all the local health departments studied, 62% hired additional staff using fund from the CDC's Preparedness Cooperative Agreement. Most local health departments have written or updated a Pandemic Flu Preparedness Plan (89%), participated in emergency drills or exercises (86%), and conducted staff training for emergency preparedness (85%). For 80% of local health departments, Emergency Operations Centers were activated in response to a natural disaster or severe weather.

Personal Health Care

Local health departments are substantially less likely to provide personal health care services. Of all the departments studied, 29% offer oral health services, 25% offer home health care, 11% offer comprehensive primary care, 9% offer behavioral and mental health services, and 7% offer substance abuse treatment services. Departments serving more than 500,000 people are more than twice as likely to offer oral health services and 3 or more times as likely to offer comprehensive primary care, behavior and mental health services, and substance abuse services than are departments serving fewer than 50,000 people. The reverse is true of home health care services, however. Departments serving populations smaller than 100,000 are more than twice as likely to offer home health care as are departments serving more than 500,000.

Most local health departments provide some treatments for communicable diseases. Of all the departments studied, 72% provide treatment for TB and 57% for STDs. Treatment for HIV/AIDS was offered by 20% of departments. Again, the likelihood that a department provides treatment services generally increases with the population size of the jurisdiction. Although only 15% of departments serving small populations offer treatment for HIV/AIDS, nearly 40% of large departments do.

FUNDING PUBLIC HEALTH

Funding for the public health system is mainly from public sources: taxes and other monies, such as fees, collected by the government at the federal, state, and local levels. The total expenditure for the public health system in 2008 is estimated by the CMS as $69.4 billion, of which $10.4 billion came from the federal government and $59 billion from state and local government (CMS, 2010). These figures do not include some important public health services:

Government spending for public works, environmental functions (air and water pollution abatement, sanitation and sewage treatment, water supplies, and so on), emergency planning and other such functions are not included. Most Federal government public health activity emanates from the Department of Health and Human Services. The Food and Drug Administration and the Centers for Disease Control account for the great majority of Federal spending in the area. Since the 9/11 catastrophe, substantial public health funding has come from two other sources: The Public Health and Social Services Emergency Fund, a part of the HHS Departmental Management Budget, and the Department of Homeland Security. State and local government public health activity expenditures are primarily for the operation of State and local health departments. Federal payments to State and local governments are deducted to avoid double counting, as are expenditures made through the Maternal and Child Health Program and the Crippled Children's Program. Disbursements made by State and local government departments for environmental functions (water and sewer authorities, for example) are not included. (CMS, 2007, p. 11)

There are many challenges to measuring public health expenditures in the United States (Sensenig, 2007). Chief among them is the difficulty of defining what government activities constitute public health services. "There is no clear-cut, universally accepted definition of government public health care services" (Sensenig, p. 103). Also, the distinction between health and public health services is not clear in the classification of budget categories. Finally, the government must collect expenditure data according to the Classification of the Functions of Government (COFOG), which is an international system developed by the United Nations.

Federal

The 2008 federal outlay for public health activities, in large categories, is contained in Table 3.3 (CMS, 2009).

The federal public health budget is used for two purposes: (a) to fund federal activities and (b) to fund state and local activities by returning federal money to states. "Most of the CDC's funding to the states is distributed

TABLE 3.3   Public Health Outlay Categories by the Federal Government, 2008

Category	Dollars (in millions)
Disease control, research, and training	$5,249
Public health and social services emergency fund	$2,529
Departmental management	$236
Food safety and inspection	$860
Food and Drug Administration	$1,514
Total	$10,388

through 'categorical grants' that are program-focused, restricted to specific program use, and do not go to support broader or core public health responsibilities. The basis for the distribution of categorical funds varies from program to program; some funds are awarded on a population basis, some on a demonstration of need, and others on a competitive basis. When taken together, funding is not necessarily determined by population or by disease burden" (Levi, Juliano, & Richardson, 2007).

Federal categorical and block grants may be criticized because they require states to engage in activities mandated by particular grant program requirements rather than in accordance with the needs of the particular population being served. That is, because federal funding is available for one kind of program, a state may dedicate resources to that program area to obtain funds, even if the program does not align with the priorities dictated by the health needs of the state. Although this is not true of every federal grant program—the Preventive Health and Health Services Block Grant mentioned earlier, for example, allows for considerable flexibility in how the funds are used—the large proportion of state health department resources that come from the federal government should be kept in mind when considering state health department budgets. In effect, not all dollars available to the state health department are created equal—they are not all part of a general pool that can be simply allocated in accordance with the state's health needs and priorities. The availability of state sources of funding may therefore be critical in financing essential services in a manner that is consistent with the state's needs and priorities.

There is wide variation in the amount of state resources expended by state public health departments.

State

As discussed previously, public health financing in the United States derives from a complex web of intergovernmental relationships at the federal, state, and local levels. Other than sharing common legal frameworks and federal funding opportunities, each state government is organized very differently with its own priorities and organizational structure when it comes to public health. As such, a comprehensive, up-to-date, and accurate summary public health financing is difficult (Sensenig, 2007; Turnock & Atchison, 2002).

For example, while California had approximately 50% more people than Texas in 2003, its government was nearly 3 times as large in terms of expenditures. However, Texas spent 4 times more on public health than

California, mostly because of the greater amount of federal funding received by Texas. Subtracting the entry of federal funds, Texas' appropriated funds were still 45% more than California and as a proportion of total state expenditures, much larger. Overall, California spent $14.7/person on population health in 2003, and Texas spent $99.3/person. Most of Texas' public health spending went for chronic disease control and support for health behavior change, using federal funds (Milbank Memorial Fund, 2005).

When trying to understand the financing of public health departments and public health activities, in particular, one should not assume that the numbers across states are comparable. Whereas Rhode Island and Hawaii have no local health departments, other states are organized with all local health departments independent from the state health departments. These differences mean per capita spending is not comparable because funding may be at the local rather than the state level or vice versa. In addition, states may differ in the amount they appropriate for public health through taxation and fees, but they may also vary in the amount of "pass-through" funding that they obtain from the federal government. On average, state population health expenditures represented 1.7% of state budgets and ranged from a low of 0.3% in California to a high of 4.4% in Montana in 2003 (Milbank Memorial Fund, 2005).

Local

Source of Local Public Health Funding

Local health departments obtain funding from a combination of sources that includes local funds, state-direct funds, federal pass-through funds such as from categorical grants, federal-direct funds, Medicaid and Medicare funds, and fees. Figure 3.2 shows the percentage of funding received from each

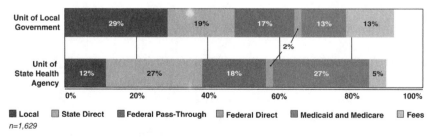

FIGURE 3.2   Mean Percentage of Total LHD Revenues from Selected Sources, by Type of LHD Governance

source for the two basic types of local health departments: (a) those that are units of local government and (b) those that are units of the state health agency. Health departments that are locally controlled obtain far less money from the state and from Medicaid and Medicare funds than departments that are units of the state. As a result, they depend more heavily on local funds and fees.

Even though control of a local health department—local or state—influences its funding sources, other factors play a role as well, because there is great heterogeneity in the funding mix for local health departments that is not explained by control. For example, although both are states where local health departments are primarily governed locally, departments in New York receive, on average, 6% of their funding from local sources, whereas Wisconsin departments receive 39% of their funds from local sources. Similarly, in both California and Missouri, departments are units of local government, but Missouri departments receive 10% of their funds directly from the state, whereas California departments get 50% of their funds from the state. Maine departments receive 59% of their revenue in federal pass-through funds, whereas Alaska departments receive 5% from the same source. Thirteen percent of funding for South Carolina departments comes directly from the federal government, whereas North Carolina departments report that 0% of their revenue is in the form of direct federal funds. Alabama departments receive 60% of their funds through Medicare and Medicaid, whereas Arizona departments receive 2% of their revenue from those sources (NACCHO, 2009). This observation is consistent with the findings of Levi et al. (2007) and the Trust for America's Future (2010), which found that the organization structure for a state health department—be it an independent agency, mixed function agency, or part of an umbrella agency—plays little role in the amount of state funding the agency receives.

Amount Expended on Local Public Health

Another issue concerning funding of local health departments is the amount spent on public health. The diversity among LHDs is clearly evident when annual budgets are examined. These ranged from less than $10,000 to more than $ 1 billion. Of all the local health departments studied, 25% had annual expenditures of under $500,000, and 17% had annual expenditures of more than $5 million. To take into account the large variation in the populations

TABLE 3.4   Mean Annual per Capita and Median Annual per Capita
Expenditures for Local Health Departments by Selected
Characteristics, 2008

LHD Characteristics	Unadjusted		Adjusted	
	Median	Mean	Median	Mean
All LHDs	$36	$64	22%	22%
Size of Population Served				
<25,000	$39	$76	26%	12%
25,000–49,999	$32	$63	25%	48%
50,000–99,999	$35	$46	23%	24%
100,000–249,999	$35	$43	11%	16%
250,000–499,999	$35	$51	9%	8%
500,000–999,999	$41	$112	12%	24%
1,000,000+	$42	$88	7%	38%
Type of Governance				
Unit of Local Government	$35	$66	17%	21%
Unit of the State Health Agency	$41	$60	39%	37%
	n = 2,097		n = 1,557	

served by local health departments, we examine per capita spending. Per
capita expenditures, again, are very variable. The typical expenditure is
about $35/capita, but the range is from less than $20 to more than $50/
capita. In general, the larger the population served, the more a local health
department spends per capita, with departments serving more than 1 million people spending on average 44% more per person than departments
serving populations of fewer than 50,000 people (see Table 3.4; NACCHO,
2009). The adjusted percentages are the percentage of unadjusted per capita expenditures accounted for by third-party payments including Medicare,
Medicaid, and private insurance, as well as patient fees. Basically, this adjustment reduces per capita expenditures for other than personal health
care (NACCHO, 2009).

There is no apparent regional pattern that explains variation. For example, states with the highest per capita expenditures include California
and New York. States with the lowest per capita expenditures include
Connecticut and Texas. Figure 3.3 shows the median annual per capita expenditure by local health departments by state.

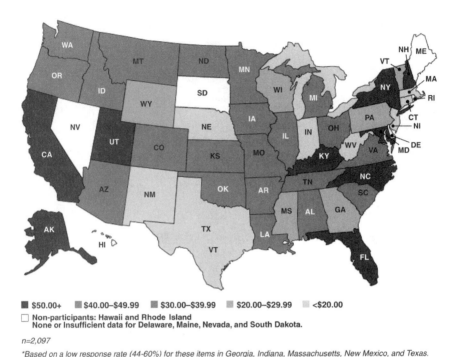

■ $50.00+   ■ $40.00–$49.99   ■ $30.00–$39.99   ■ $20.00–$29.99   ▢ <$20.00
▢ Non-participants: Hawaii and Rhode Island
None or Insufficient data for Delaware, Maine, Nevada, and South Dakota.

n=2,097

*Based on a low response rate (44-60%) for these items in Georgia, Indiana, Massachusetts, New Mexico, and Texas.

FIGURE 3.3   Median Annual per Capita LHD Expenditures, by State*

Other Funding Consideration

Federal, state, and local expenditures do not tell the entire story of public health spending in local areas.

Measuring investments in public health, particularly in Essential Services, in a given jurisdiction must go well beyond measuring only local health department expenditures. The health status and well-being of a community is a function of the collective efforts of many 'community partners,' including the health department, other social and human service agencies, primary care providers, hospitals, businesses, community groups, schools, churches, volunteer organizations, and the citizenry itself. The relative contributions of these entities varies considerably from community to community, depending on a host of factors, including geography, political imperatives, the local economy, market forces, and public health infrastructure. (Barry, Centra, Pratt, Carol, & Giordano, 1998, p. 31)

REFERENCES

Association of State and Territorial Health Officials. (2008). *2007 State public health workforce survey results.* Arlington, VA: Author.

Association of State and Territorial Health Officials. (2009). *Profile of state public health, volume one.* Arlington, VA: Author.

Baker, E. L., & Koplan, J. P. (2002). Strengthening the nation's public health infrastructure: Historic challenge, unprecedented opportunity. *Health Affairs, 21,* 15–27.

Baker, E. L., Potter, M. A., Jones, D. L., Mercer, S. L., Cioffi, J. P., Green, L. W., et al. (2005). The public health infrastructure and our nation's health. *Annual Review of Public Health, 26,* 303–318.

Barry, M. A., Centra L., Pratt E. T. B. Jr, Carol, K., & Giordano, L. (1998). *Where do the dollars go? Measuring local public health expenditures.* A report submitted by the National Association of County and City Health Officials, the National Association of Local Boards of Health, and the Public Health Foundation to the Office of Disease Prevention and Health Promotion, Office of Public Health and Science, U.S. Department of Health and Human Services.

Bavier, A. R. (2009). Agency for Healthcare Research and Quality. *Encyclopedia of Health Services Research* in Ross M. Mullner, Editor, Thousand Oaks, CA: Sage Publications pp. 38–41.

Beitsch, L. M., Brooks, R. G., Grigg, M., & Menachemi, N. (2006). Structure and functions of state public health agencies. *American Journal of Public Health, 96,* 167–172.

Centers for Disease Control and Prevention. (2007). *National public health performance standards user guide.* Retrieved July 1, 2010, from, http://www. cdc.gov/od/ocphp/nphpsp/PDF/UserGuide.pdf

Centers for Medicare & Medicaid Services. (2007). *National health expenditures accounts: Definitions, sources, and methods, 2008.* Retrieved July 20, 2010, from https://www.cms.gov/NationalHealthExpendData/downloads/dsm-08.pdf

Centers for Medicare & Medicaid Services. (2010). *National Health Expenditure Data, Historical.* Retrieved July 20, 2010, from http://www.cms.gov/NationalHealthExpendData/downloads/tables.pdf

Centers for Medicare & Medicaid Services, Office of the Actuary, National Health Statistics Group. (2009). *Budget of the United States Government: Detailed functional tables, fiscal year 2008: Table 25–13: Current services budget authority by function, category and program.* Retrieved July 20, 2010, from http://www.gpoaccess.gov/usbudget/fy08/fct.html

Committee on Assuring the Health of the Public in the 21st Century. (2002.). *The future of the public's health in the 21st century.* Washington DC: National Academy Press.

Fee, E., & Brown, T. M. (2002). The unfulfilled promise of public health: Déjà vu all over again. *Health Affairs, 21*, 31–43.

Hartsaw, K. (2009). Centers for Disease Control and Prevention. *Encyclopedia of Health Services Research* in Ross M. Mullner, Editor. Thousand Oaks, CA: Sage Publications pp. 141–144

Health Resources and Services Administration, Bureau of Primary Health Care. (2010). *The health center program: What is a health center?* Retrieved October 25, 2010 from http://bphc.hrsa.gov/about/

Institute of Medicine. (1988). *The future of public health.* Washington, DC: National Academy Press.

Institute of Medicine. (2003). *The future of the public's health in the 21st century.* Washington, DC: National Academies Press.

Levi, J., Juliano, C., & Richardson, M. (2007). Financing public health: Diminished funding for core needs and state-by-state variation in support. *Journal of Public Health Management and Practice, 13*, 97–102.

Mays, G. P., Beitsch, L. M., Corso, L., Chang, C., & Brewer, R. (2007). States gathering momentum: Promising strategies for accreditation and assessment activities in multistate learning collaborative applicant states. *Journal of Public Health Management and Practice, 13*, 364–373.

Mays, G. P., McHugh, M. C., Shim, K., Perry, N., Lenaway, D., Halverson, P. K., et al. (2006). Institutional and economic determinants of public health system performance. *American Journal of Public Health, 96*, 523–531.

McCarty, K. L., Nelson, G. D., Hodge, J. G., & Gebbie, K. M. (2009). Major components and themes of local public health laws in select U.S. jurisdictions. *Public Health Reports, 124*, 458–462.

Milbank Memorial Fund. (2005). *2002–2003 State health expenditure report.* New York: Author.

National Association of County and City Health Officials. (2009). *2008 National profile of local health departments.* Washington, DC: Author.

National Association of County and City Health Officials. (2010). *The local health department workforce: Findings from the 2008 national profile of local health departments.* Washington, DC: Author.

National Center for Health Statistics. (2010a). *About the National Center for Health Statistics.* Retrieved July 20, 2010, from http://www.cdc.gov/nchs/about.htm

National Center for Health Statistics. (2010b). *Surveys and data collection systems.* Retrieved July 20, 2010, from http://www.cdc.gov/nchs/surveys.htm

Passenger Cases. (1849) 48 U.S. 283, 414.

Perlino, C. M. (2006). *Medicaid, prevention, and public health: Invest today for a healthier tomorrow.* Washington, DC: American Public Health Association.

Public Health Functions Steering Committee, Office of Disease Prevention and Health Promotion, Office of Public Health and Science, U.S. Department of Health and Human Services. (1994). *Public health in America.* Washington, DC: U.S. Department of Health and Human Services.

Sensenig, A. L. (2007). Refining estimates of public health spending as measured in national health expenditures accounts: The United States experience. *Journal of Public Health Management and Practice, 13,* 103–114.

Tilson, H., & Berkowitz, B. (2006). The public health enterprise: Examining our twenty-first-century policy challenges. *Health Affairs, 25,* 900–910.

Trust for America's Future. (2010). *Shortchanging America's health.* Washington, DC: Author.

Turnock, B. J., & Atchison, C. (2002). Governmental public health in the United States: The implications of federalism. *Health Affairs, 21,* 68–78.

U.S. Department of Veterans Affairs. (2010). *Medical centers.* Retrieved July 20, 2010, from http://www1.va.gov/health/MedicalCenters.asp

U.S. Department of Health and Human Services. (2000). *Healthy People 2010* (2nd ed.). With understanding and improving health and objectives for improving health (2 vols.). Washington, DC: U.S. Government Printing Office.

U.S. Department of Health and Human Services. (2009). *Fiscal year 2010 budget in brief.* Washington, DC: U.S. Government Printing Office.

U.S. Department of Health and Human Services. (2010a). *HHS: About us.* Retrieved July 20, 2010, from http://www.hhs.gov/ab out/

U.S. Department of Health and Human Services. (2010b). *HHS: What we do.* Retrieved July 20, 2010, from http://www.hhs.gov/about/whatwedo.html

U.S. Department of Health and Human Services. (2010c). *Fiscal year 2010 budget in brief.* Retrieved July 20, 2010, from http://dhhs.gov/asfr/ob/docbudget/2010budgetinbrief.pdf

Van Wave, T. W., Scutchfield, F. D., & Honoré, P. A. (2010). Recent advances in public health systems research in the United States. *Annual Review of Public Health, 31,* 283–295.

4

Infectious Disease Control

Infectious disease control continues to be an essential part of public health in the United States and throughout the world. In the mid-20th century, some believed that infectious diseases were a health problem of the past. We now know that this is not true. As Moore (2007) expressively puts it:

> The word "plague" would have sent a ripple of fear down the spines of the people in (Shakespeare's) audiences, and the fact that they had no knowledge of the agent that swept invisibly across continents, devastating populations and leaving families shattered and entire economies in tatters, only served to heighten the anxiety.
>
> We have come a long way since Shakespeare's sixteenth century. We know about bacteria, viruses, and microscopic protozoa. We can watch the way that these tiny agents move into our bodies and damage our organs. We have a growing understanding of how our body mounts defensive strategies that fight off these invaders, and have built some clever chemical that can help mount an assault on these bio-villains. In the middle of the twentieth century, as science was creating a new optimism, some serious commentators believed that the total eradication of nasty bacteria and viruses could be just a decade or so away. But it wasn't. Far from it. (p. 6)

Today, both primary and secondary prevention are important public health practices related to infectious disease control. As will be evident, the methods used for primary prevention include the classic surveillance, sanitation, vaccination, and quarantine. Treatment relies on providing antimicrobial drug therapy and developing new therapies in response to new strains as well as antimicrobial resistance among existing strains. Although the methods for preventing and treating infectious diseases are, in general, the same as in the past, great improvements in these methods have resulted because of advances in microbiology, information and communication systems, and laboratory techniques. Following are descriptions of public health practice related to five infectious disease problems today: pandemic and avian influenza, perinatal hepatitis B, foodborne diseases, and childhood vaccinations.

PANDEMIC AND AVIAN INFLUENZA

Pandemic influenza, by definition, is a *global public health emergency*. There is no human disease that causes more illness and death in a matter of months than an outbreak of pandemic flu. An influenza pandemic is a rare but recurring event and significantly different from avian influenza and seasonal influenza. Avian influenza refers to many different types of influenza viruses that primarily affect birds and, on rare occasions, these avian viruses may affect other species including humans. The rapid expansion of avian H5N1 influenza from Asia to Europe, and now Africa may or may not adapt into a strain that is readily contagious among humans. If this rare adaptation occurs and it crosses species from birds to humans, it will then become a human influenza disease (Taubenberger et al., 2005; Tumpey et al., 2005). Seasonal influenza occurs each and every year with some variation and causes approximately 36,000 deaths annually in the United States alone. There is a vaccine available each year, which may prevent or ameliorate illness in the majority of people infected. Whether there are large numbers of deaths from pandemic influenza is determined primarily by four factors:

- Number of people infected;
- Virulence of the virus;
- Vulnerability of the affected populations; and
- Effectiveness of preventive measures, such as isolation, quarantine, antiviral medications, and vaccines if available.

The social and economic disruption in all countries affected can be tremendous. High rates of absenteeism in the workplace and in schools can be expected, as well as significant disruption in essential services and supplies of food, transportation, education, communications, and energy.

Global influenza pandemics are rare but have occurred on three occasions in the past century. In 1918, the Spanish influenza pandemic killed an estimated 50 million people worldwide (see Figure 4.1). It is believed by many to have caused more illness and death than any other disease in human history. A second influenza pandemic, known as the Asian influenza (H2N2), occurred in 1957. It resulted in an estimated 2 million deaths worldwide. A third pandemic in 1968, known as the Hong Kong influenza

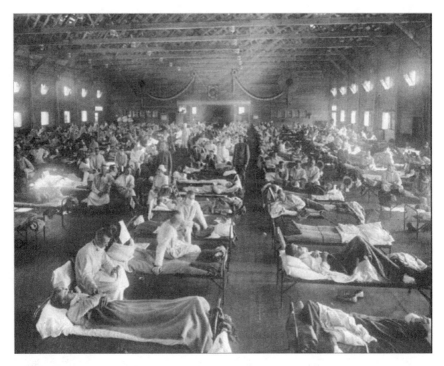

FIGURE 4.1   In 1918, influenza victims crowded into an emergency hospital at Fort Riley in Kansas. From the National Museum of Health and Medicine, Armed Forces Institute of Pathology.

(H3N2), killed more than 1 million people. Influenza pandemics are *rare* but *recurrent* events that meet three criteria:

- Result from a new influenza virus that emerges in a population that has little or *no* immunity,
- Cause *serious* illness and death in humans, and
- Require *sustained* human-to-human transmission by respiratory droplet (i.e., by coughing and sneezing).

Avian Influenza

As highly pathogenic avian influenza A/H5N1 races across the continents from Asia to Europe, and now to Africa and the Middle East, the H5N1 pathogen has resulted in the death of more than 150 million birds—the largest and most severe case on record. The risk of human infection from the H5N1 avian virus persists as long as opportunities for direct contact exist between humans and infected birds. The risk from direct infection from H5N1 in birds occurs when the virus passes directly from infected poultry via feces to humans and may result in serious illness or death. As the number of confirmed human cases of avian influenza A/H5N1 in the world approaches 200, the mortality rate remains more than 50%. As the contact between infected birds and humans continues, the potential for the admixing of avian and human viral components increases. A pandemic influenza in humans *may* or *may not* occur as the result of the avian influenza outbreak over the last 9 years. Nevertheless, the danger of it happening exists.

The avian influenza virus can improve its transmissibility among humans through two primary mechanisms (Belshe, 2005):

- An explosive outbreak and surge of cases can occur in humans when there is a *reassortment of genetic material* between avian and human viruses in humans or in another species such as swine. This could result in a rapidly transmissible pandemic outbreak of influenza in humans.
- A second mechanism is the more gradual process of *adaptive, mutational change* of the avian virus that may bind to human cells and increase human infections. This may result in subsequent and more gradual outbreaks of human-to-human transmission of influenza.

There is the risk that the H5N1 avian virus, which is circulating widely among birds in many continents today, may develop the characteristics needed to begin another influenza pandemic. To date, it has met all the prerequisites for the beginning of a pandemic except the ability to spread in a sustained manner from person-to-person. Therefore, although there is the possibility that a pandemic influenza in humans may not occur, the probability decreases as the spread of avian influenza virus continues.

The most recently confirmed cases of avian influenza A/H5N1 have identified direct contact with infected birds as the most likely source of exposure. To date, the World Health Organization (WHO) has reported human cases in seven countries: Cambodia, China, Indonesia, Thailand, Vietnam, Iraq, and Turkey. All human cases have occurred in countries where highly pathogenic avian influenza has been found in poultry. There is one reported case of probable human-to-human transmission in Thailand in September 2004. No evidence of sustained human-to-human transmission of H5N1 has been detected, although rare instances of probable human-to-human transmission have occurred (Ungchusak et al., 2005).

Because there is no evidence of sustained human-to-human transmission of the virus occurring in any country, simply traveling to an outbreak country does not place an individual at risk of infection, provided the person does not have very close or direct contact with diseased birds in these countries. A history of poultry consumption in an affected country is not a risk factor if the food is thoroughly cooked and the person was not involved in any food preparation. In areas with avian influenza and confirmed human cases, poultry can be safely consumed if properly cooked and handled during preparation. The H5N1 virus is sensitive to heat, and normal cooking temperatures will kill the virus. However, cross-contamination from juices of raw poultry products during food preparation can transmit the virus, and there should be no mixing of any items or eating of any raw poultry products. Persons involved in food preparation should thoroughly wash their hands and clean surfaces in contact with poultry products with soap and water. Raw eggs should not be used in foods that will not be heat-treated by cooking or baking in these outbreak areas. Avian influenza virus is *not* transmitted through cooked food and clinical investigations to date have shown no evidence that anyone has become infected following the consumption of properly cooked poultry or egg products.

Clinical Manifestations

In the confirmed human cases of avian influenza A/H5N1, the disease followed an unusually aggressive clinical course with rapid deterioration and a mortality rate of more than 50%. The incubation period for H5N1 avian influenza in humans may be longer than the normal seasonal influenza incubation period of 2–3 days and may last 8 days or longer. Initial signs and symptoms include high fever (greater than 38°C) and influenza-like respiratory symptoms. It may be accompanied by watery diarrhea, vomiting, abdominal pain, chest pain, and bleeding from the nose, or, in rare instances, lack of respiratory symptoms that present as acute encephalitis. In many patients, a rapid clinical deterioration has been accompanied by multi-organ failure. Laboratory abnormalities include leukopenia, lymphopenia, thrombocytopenia, liver function abnormalities, and, in some cases, a disseminated intravascular coagulation. The U.S. Food and Drug Administration (USFDA) cleared the only laboratory method for diagnostic testing of avian influenza A/H5 (Asian lineage) by real-time reverse transcription-polymerase chain reaction (RT-PCR; CDC, 2006a). Testing for this virus is indicated when a patient has a severe respiratory illness and a risk of exposure to dead, ill, or infected poultry in a country with outbreaks of influenza H5N1 among poultry.

Limited evidence suggests that oseltamivir (Tamiflu), a neuramini-dase inhibitor, can improve the prospects of survival if administered within 48 hours of symptom onset. However, with relatively few clinical cases to date, it is difficult to determine the effectiveness of antiviral medications. Unfortunately, most cases have occurred in *children* and *young adults* and have been detected and treated late in the course of illness. Recommendations on the optimum dose and treatment for avian influenza A/H5N1 in adults and children are currently undergoing review because these cases may require an increased duration of treatment.

Planning and Preparedness

The WHO's Global Influenza Surveillance Network (GISN) is a critical component of preparedness throughout the world for pandemic influenza. The GISN:

. . . enables WHO to recommend twice annually the content of the influenza vaccine for the subsequent influenza season. More than 250 million doses of influenza vaccine are produced annually which contain the WHO recommended influenza strains.

Frequent updating of the influenza vaccine content is necessary as influenza viruses are permanently evolving. Only a vaccine whose virus strains match the circulating influenza viruses will protect recipients efficiently from influenza disease and death.

The WHO Influenza Surveillance Network serves also as a global alert mechanism for the emergence of influenza viruses with pandemic potential. Its activities have contributed greatly to the understanding of influenza epidemiology. The network was established in 1952, after a WHO Expert Committee recommended that through an international network of laboratories, WHO would be able to advise WHO Member States as to "what influenza control measures are useful, useless or harmful". . . . The main components of the WHO Global Influenza Surveillance Network are National Influenza Centres (NICs) which sample patients with influenza-like-illness and submit representative isolates to WHO Collaborating Centres (WHO CCs) for antigenic and genetic analyses. NICs, WHO CCs and WHO form the WHO Global Influenza Surveillance Network, with collaboration based on agreed terms of reference.

Currently, 134 institutions from 104 countries are recognized by WHO as National Influenza Centres. In addition, various other laboratories have regularly submitted influenza viruses to the Programme in the past years. (WHO, 2010)

The United States has four WHO National Influenza Centers: the Viral and Rickettsial Disease Laboratory in California; the School of Public Health, Department of Epidemiology in Ann Arbor, Michigan; the Centers for Disease Control and Prevention (CDC) in Georgia; and the Virology Diagnostic Services Laboratory of Zoonotic Diseases at the Wadsworth Center in New York.

As the countries of the world, including the United States, plan for pandemic influenza, preparedness efforts revolve around the following:

- Enhanced surveillance and early identification of cases in humans with isolation and contact tracing, and quarantine for exposed individuals to decrease transmission to others;
- Communication and education of health care professionals and the public about the seriousness of the situation;
- Implementation of infection control measures and the provision of quality medical and supportive care;
- Maintenance of emergency and essential community services; and
- Outbreak control via the use of antiviral treatments, prophylaxis, and vaccination, if available.

Local health departments have been planning for a pandemic flu for several years. In recent years, there has also been greater collaboration between local health departments and other local governmental departments as part of overall disaster preparedness. This has allowed the departments of health to work more closely with the police, fire, rescue, and emergency services, local hospitals and physicians, and various other public safety units. It is believed that any major effort to respond to this threat will require a strong local response.

To respond to a pandemic influenza, vaccine manufacturers need the capability to develop and produce large quantities of new vaccines within months and not the 8 to 10 years that is needed today. This will entail making huge investments in new technologies to produce vaccines rapidly. Developing a cell-culture–derived vaccine instead of depending on chicken egg embryos, creating a library of clinical grade vaccine strains that are now appearing, new microdiagnostic laboratory assays, refining production methods to reduce the time and cost of making vaccines, and boosting an immune response after a single dose of a nasal spray vaccine would all be major contributions to an effective response to a pandemic influenza. Traditional public health methods to control an outbreak may include isolation and quarantine of infected persons, which may be ineffective after a short period.

Recent literature raised important questions regarding the implication of resistance to antiviral agents for the management of influenza and for planning a response to a possible pandemic (Hayden, 2006). Because of the high levels of resistance to amantadine and rimantadine detected among influenza A viruses, the CDC recommended in 2006 that neither drug be used for the treatment or chemoprophylaxis of influenza A infections (CDC, 2006b). Given that the two most important medical interventions— vaccines and antiviral medications—may likely be in short supply, federal, state, and local efforts need a strong community education program on methods of infection control. It is recommended that all communities be targeted for infection control education, including minority, low-income, and immigrant populations.

Public health officials believe that it is of paramount importance that federal and state level governments invest in the local infrastructure. Appropriate activities include enhanced funding for local medical research institutions, local hospitals, physicians, nurses, educators and other professionals, and devoting substantial resources to local emergency and public health systems. Pandemic influenza is rare, but the probability of it reoccurring is increasing. When pandemic influenza does occur, it will probably cause more illness and death in a shorter time frame than any other public health threat currently being faced.

PERINATAL HEPATITIS B

A major component of the public health effort to prevent infectious disease outbreaks is the CDC's National Notifiable Diseases Surveillance System (NNDSS). The history of this program begins in the 19th century:

> In 1878, Congress authorized the U.S. Marine Hospital Service (i.e., the forerunner of the Public Health Service [PHS]) to collect morbidity reports regarding cholera, smallpox, plague, and yellow fever from U.S. consuls overseas; this information was to be used for instituting quarantine measures to prevent the introduction and spread of these diseases into the United States. In 1879, a specific Congressional appropriation was made for the collection and publication of reports of these notifiable diseases. The authority for weekly reporting and publication

of these reports was expanded by Congress in 1893 to include data from states and municipal authorities. To increase the uniformity of the data, Congress enacted a law in 1902 directing the Surgeon General to provide forms for the collection and compilation of data and for the publication of reports at the national level. In 1912, state and territorial health authorities—in conjunction with PHS—recommended immediate telegraphic reporting of five infectious diseases and the monthly reporting, by letter, of 10 additional diseases. The first annual summary of The Notifiable Diseases in 1912 included reports of 10 diseases from 19 states, the District of Columbia, and Hawaii. By 1928, all states, the District of Columbia, Hawaii, and Puerto Rico were participating in national reporting of 29 specified diseases. At their annual meeting in 1950, the State and Territorial Health Officers authorized a conference of state and territorial epidemiologists whose purpose was to determine which diseases should be reported to PHS. In 1961, CDC assumed responsibility for the collection and publication of data concerning nationally notifiable diseases (CDC, 2010d)

The NNDSS collects data from state and local authorities about selected notifiable infectious diseases. The states report cases to the CDC voluntarily. Currently, reporting is mandated only at the state level through state legislation or regulation. In general, all states report the internationally quarantinable diseases, which include cholera, plague, and yellow fever, to comply with the WHO's International Health Regulations. The CDC, in collaboration with the Council of State and Territorial Epidemiologists (CSTE), updates the list of reportable diseases annually. The CDC published Case Definitions for Public Health Surveillance in 1990, providing uniform criteria for reporting cases for the first time and including infectious and noninfectious diseases. The results of the NNDSS are published weekly in the *Morbidity and Mortality Weekly Report* (*MMWR*) and annually in a year-end summary. See the 2010 list of notifiable infectious and noninfectious diseases in Table 4.1 (CDC, 2010d).

One of the notifiable infectious diseases monitored by the NNDSS is hepatitis B. The hepatitis B virus (HBV) infection is an established cause of acute and chronic hepatitis and cirrhosis. It is the cause of up to 80% of hepatocellular carcinoma and is second only to tobacco among known human carcinogens. More than 350,000 million persons are chronically infected worldwide, and there were 600,000 deaths in 2002 from hepatitis B infection. The virus is transmitted through blood or other bodily fluids,

TABLE 4.1   Nationally Notifiable Diseases, 2010

Infectious Diseases

Anthrax
Arboviral neuroinvasive and nonneuroinvasive diseases (such as West Nile)
Botulism
Brucellosis
Chancroid
Chlamydia trachomatis infection
Cholera
Cryptosporidiosis
Cyclosporiasis
Dengue
Diphtheria
Ehrlichiosis/Anaplasmosis
Giardiasis
Gonorrhea
Haemophilus influenzae, invasive disease
Hansen disease (leprosy)
Hantavirus pulmonary syndrome
Hemolytic uremic syndrome, postdiarrheal
Hepatitis (A, B, and C)
HIV infection
Influenza-associated pediatric mortality
Legionellosis
Listeriosis
Lyme disease
Malaria
Measles
Meningococcal disease
Mumps
Novel influenza A virus infections
Pertussis
Plague
Poliomyelitis, paralytic
Poliovirus infection, nonparalytic
Psittacosisa
Q Fever
Rabies

Rubella
Rubella, congenital syndrome
Salmonellosis
Severe acute respiratory syndrome-associated coronavirus (SARS-CoV) disease
Shiga toxin-producing *Escherichia coli* (STEC)
Shigellosis
Smallpox
Spotted fever rickettsiosis
Streptococcal toxic-shock syndrome
Streptococcus pneumoniae, invasive disease
Syphilis
Tetanus
Toxic-shock syndrome (other than Streptococcal)
Trichinellosis (Trichinosis)
Tuberculosis
Tularemia
Typhoid fever
Vancomycin-intermediate *Staphylococcus aureus* (VISA)
Vancomycin-resistant *Staphylococcus aureus* (VRSA)
Varicella (morbidity)
Varicella (deaths only)
Vibriosis
Viral hemorrhagic fevers (such as Ebola and Marburg)
Yellow fever

Non-infectious Diseases

Cancer
Elevated blood lead levels
Pesticide-related illness, acute
Silicosis
Waterborne disease outbreak

Source: National Notifiable Diseases Surveillance System, CDC, 2010d

and it is 50–100 times more infectious than HIV. Approximately 10% of all acute HBV infections progress to chronic infection with the risk of chronic HBV infection decreasing with age. As many as 90% of infants who acquire HBV infection from their mothers at birth become chronically infected, or carriers. Of children who become infected with HBV between 1 and 5 years of age, 30%–50% become carriers. Persons with chronic HBV infection are often asymptomatic and may not be aware that they are infected, yet are capable of infecting others. About 25% of adults who become carriers as children die from liver cancer or cirrhosis caused by the infection. Chronic infection is responsible for most HBV-related morbidity and mortality, including chronic hepatitis, cirrhosis, liver failure, and hepatocellular carcinoma. Persons with chronic HBV infection are at 12–300 times higher risk of hepatocellular carcinoma than noncarriers (CDC, 2009c; WHO, 2010).

The hepatitis B vaccine is safe and effective according to the WHO and has been available in the United States since 1981. Since then, the control of perinatal infection has been a crucial part of the evolving vaccination strategy of the Advisory Committee on Immunization Practices (ACIP). The CDC, American Academy of Pediatrics (AAP), and the ACIP recommend maternal identification through screening and newborn prophylaxis, which can significantly reduce neonatal infection and potential sequelae.

Preventing perinatal HBV transmission is an integral part of the national strategy to eliminate Hepatitis B in the United States. National guidelines call for the following:

■ Universal screening of pregnant women for HBsAg during each pregnancy,
■ Case management of HBsAg-positive mothers and their infants,
■ Provision of immunoprophylaxis for infants born to infected mothers, including Hepatitis B vaccine and Hepatitis B immune globulin [sic],
■ Routine vaccination of all infants with the Hepatitis B vaccine series, with the first dose administered at birth (CDC, 2010b)

To accomplish the goal of eliminating perinatal hepatitis B transmission, many local health departments administer the Perinatal Hepatitis B Prevention Program in coordination with the CDC (CDC, 2010g).

Public Health Management: Case of New York State

New York State Public Health Law requires the completion of the following steps if a pregnant woman is hepatitis B surface antigen (HBsAg)–positive:

Reporting of the Case

- Physicians report to the County Department of Health's Perinatal Hepatitis B Prevention Program.
- Diagnostic laboratories report to the County Department of Health's Perinatal Hepatitis B Prevention Program.
- Labor and delivery hospitals report to the County Department of Health's Perinatal Hepatitis B Prevention Program.
- County Department of Health reports to New York State Department of Health (NYSDOH).

Management of the Case

- *Isolation.* Blood, body fluid, and tissue precautions are indicated for a pregnant woman who is HBsAg-positive and for her infant.
- *Investigation.* Case investigations are performed to determine the source of infection and exposure to the infant, sexual, needle sharing, and household contacts.
- *Laboratory Work and Follow-up.* Follow-up is needed regarding HBsAg status of the mother and her infant, including follow-up laboratory work to determine the success of treatment for infants who complete the hepatitis B vaccine series.
- *Counseling.* HBsAg-positive individuals shall be counseled in measures to prevent the spread of hepatitis B transmission to household, sexual, and needle-sharing contacts.
- *Referral.* Individuals diagnosed as hepatitis B carriers should be referred to their private physicians for disease management.

Management of the Contacts

- *Investigation.* Case investigation is performed to determine the exposure to household, sexual, and needle-sharing contacts.
- *Laboratory Testing and Follow-up.* Identified household, sexual, and needle-sharing contacts should be tested for the presence of HBV and vaccine offered if indicated by their physicians.
- *Infants.* The purpose of maternal screening and intervention is to prevent the development of hepatitis B infection among infants born to mothers who are HBsAg-positive.

FOODBORNE DISEASE

Foodborne disease remains a serious public health problem in the United States and worldwide.

The Council for Agricultural Science and Technology, a private non-profit organization, estimated in its 1994 report, Foodborne Pathogens: Risks and Consequences, that as many as 9,000 deaths and 6.5 to 33 million illnesses in the United States each year are food-related. Hospitalization costs alone for these illnesses are estimated at over $3 billion a year. Costs for lost productivity for seven specific pathogens have been estimated to range between $6 billion and $9 billion. Total costs for all foodborne illnesses are likely to be much higher. These estimates do not take into account the total burden placed on society by the chronic, often life-long consequences caused by some foodborne pathogens.

Additional important safety concerns are associated with the greater susceptibility to foodborne infections of several population groups. These include persons with lowered immunity due to HIV/AIDS, those on medications for cancer treatment or for organ transplantation, as well as pregnant women (and their fetuses), young children, and elderly persons. Patients taking antibiotics, or antacids, are also at greater risk of infection from some pathogens. Other groups who may be disproportionately affected include persons living in institutional settings, such as hospitals and nursing homes, and those with inadequate access to health care, such as homeless persons, migrant farm workers, and others of low socioeconomic status. (Occupational Safety and Health Administration [OSHA], 2010)

Among outbreaks for which etiology was determined in recent years, bacterial pathogens caused 75% of the outbreaks and of these, *Salmonella enteritides* was responsible for 86% of them. Chemical agents caused 17% of the outbreaks and 1% of cases; viruses, 6% of outbreaks and 8% of cases; and parasites, 2% of outbreaks, and 5% of cases. These illnesses primarily affect elderly, very young, and immunocompromised individuals. Increased travel and global trade may increase the risk of contracting and spreading foodborne illnesses.

A foodborne disease outbreak is the occurrence of two or more cases of a similar illness resulting from the ingestion of a common food. Food poisoning ranks second only to the common cold as the most frequent cause of short-term illness. Infections transmitted through the consumption of food may cause acute gastroenteritis food poisoning or various syndromes with systemic manifestations. Food poisoning is defined as the occurrence of nausea, vomiting, diarrhea, and acute gastroenteritis of short duration due to the in-gestion of food contaminated by microorganism or their products, chemical toxins, or toxic substances present naturally in certain foods. This definition includes both food intoxication and food infection. Sometimes the term *food poisoning* is limited to food intoxication.

Food may be infected at its source during manufacture, preparation, storage, and distribution. Diseases that occur at the source include trichino-sis, brucellosis, and salmonellosis.

In 2006, there was a nationwide outbreak of Shiga toxin-producing *Escherichia coli* O157:H7 enteritis linked to the consumption of contaminated leafy green vegetables (specifically spinach) from one California supplier. This was the 26th reported outbreak of *E. coli* infection in the United States that had been traced to contaminated leafy green vegetables since 1993. Each year, approximately 110,000 people acquire toxigenic *E. coli* infection, and about 50 of them die (Maki, 2006).

Foodborne illnesses can be caused by many microorganisms including bacteria, fungi, and viruses and their related toxins, parasites, and chemical contaminants. During the last 20 years, some foods that have been linked to outbreaks include milk (*Campylobacter*); unpasteurized apple cider (*E. coli* O157:H7); raw and undercooked eggs (*Salmonella*); shellfish (*Noroviruses*); fish (ciguatera poisoning); raspberries (*Cyclospora*); strawberries (hepatitis A virus); and ready-to-eat meats (*Listeria*). Only a small percentage of the people who have foodborne illnesses actually seek medical care. The bacterial agents most often identified in patients with foodborne illness in the United States are *Campylobacter*, *Salmonella*, and *Shigella*. Testing for viruses that may cause diarrheal disease is rarely done in clinical practice, even though they are considered the most common cause of foodborne illness.

Signs and Symptoms of Foodborne Illness

Foodborne illnesses typically present with gastrointestinal symptoms such as vomiting, diarrhea, and abdominal pain. However, nonspecific and neu-rological symptoms may also occur. A high degree of suspicion by the physi-cian and asking the appropriate questions may be the only opportunity to make an early clinical diagnosis of a foodborne illness. Important clues to determining the etiology of a foodborne disease are:

- Incubation period;
- Duration of illness;

- Predominant clinical symptoms; and
- Population involved.

When considering foodborne illness in the differential diagnosis, patients are asked if they have consumed raw or poorly cooked foods (e.g., eggs, meats, shellfish, fish, unpasteurized milk or juices, home-canned goods, fresh produce, or soft cheeses). They are also asked if any of their family members or close friends have similar symptoms. Questions to the patient address occupation, food preparation habits, foreign travel, contact with a farm or pet, camping, untreated water consumption, and picnic attendance. If foodborne illness is suspected, specimens are submitted for laboratory testing and the local health department is contacted. Because infectious diarrhea can be very contagious and is easily spread, rapid identification of an etiologic agent may help control disease outbreak and prevent further exposures. Deliberate contamination is a rare event, but it has been documented in the past. Intentional contamination of a food product may be suggested by the presence of an unusual pathogen in a common food, or a common agent affecting an unusually large number of people, or a common agent that is not usually seen in clinical practice, as might occur with chemical poisonings.

The following signs or symptoms may suggest the presence of a foodborne illness and laboratory testing may provide important diagnostic clues, especially in the very young, the elderly, and the immunocompromised: bloody diarrhea, weight loss, diarrhea and dehydration, fever, prolonged diarrhea over several days, neurological involvement such as paresthesias, motor weakness, cranial nerve palsies, sudden onset of nausea, vomiting or diarrhea, and severe abdominal pain. In addition to foodborne causes, a differential diagnosis should include underlying medical conditions such as inflammatory bowel diseases, malignancies, medication use, recent surgery or radiation, malabsorption syndromes, immune deficiencies, and other morbidities.

Stool cultures are indicated if the patient is febrile, has bloody diarrhea, has severe abdominal pain, or if the illness is severe or persistent in a vulnerable person. Stool cultures are also recommended if many fecal leukocytes are present. This may indicate diffuse colonic inflammation and is suggestive of invasive bacteria such as *Shigella, Salmonella, Campylobacter* and invasive *E. coli.*

Treating Foodborne Illness

Acute gastroenteritis may be self-limiting and may only require hydration and supportive care. Routine use of antidiarrheal agents is not recommended because many of these agents have potentially serious adverse effects in infants and young children. Choice of antimicrobial therapy should be based on clinical signs and symptoms, organisms present, susceptibility tests, and appropriateness of treating with an antibiotic. Table 4.2 summarizes selected common bacterial foodborne illnesses by etiology, incubation period, signs and symptoms, duration of illness, associated foods, laboratory testing, and treatment (CDC, 2004).

Selected Common Bacterial Foodborne Illnesses

The diagnosis, management, and reporting of foodborne illnesses by physicians to the local health department may identify an outbreak in the community and lead to the prevention of further cases and the removal of contaminated products from the market place. It also provides an opportunity to correct inadequate food preparation practices by establishments and to educate individuals about proper food handling practices. This is especially important with food workers who are at high risk of transmitting the disease to others.

Prevention of Foodborne Disease

The huge burden of disease from foodborne diseases—affecting thousands of people and causing many deaths—occurs despite intensive prevention efforts by the federal food safety agencies: the United States Department of Agriculture (USDA), the USFDA, and the CDC. Physicians and other health care professionals play a critical role in the prevention and control of food-related disease outbreaks because of the opportunity to identify suspicious symptoms, disease clusters, and etiological agents and report their findings to public health authorities, where they will become part of the larger network of information that monitors foodborne diseases. Specifically, physicians should recognize the potential for foodborne etiology in a patient's illness, and realize that many but not all cases of foodborne illness have gastrointestinal symptoms. They should obtain stool cultures in appropriate settings and recognize that some specific pathogens (e.g., *E. coli* O157:H7) must be requested. Physicians should talk with their patients about ways to prevent food-related diseases. They should also appreciate that any patient with a foodborne illness may represent the sentinel case of a more extensive outbreak, and therefore, it is important to understand the cause of the outbreak and to prevent its spread.

Today in the United States, virtually all food consumed is grown and processed on vast farming and industrial scales or is increasingly imported from other countries, including milk and other dairy products, eggs and egg products, fresh vegetables and fruits, and processed snacks and other food stuffs. These aspects of food delivery make prevention of foodborne diseases more difficult. Relatively little of our fresh food is now grown locally. The risk of foodborne disease is considerably higher with more food prepared outside of the home than meals made at home. The risk of diseases such as *Salmonella*, pathogenic *E. coli*, *Campylobacter*, and *Listeria* increase with centralized production and distribution of commercially produced foods, and the failure to remove bacterial contaminants in a single production step can result in a shipment of contaminated food to millions of consumers.

Efforts to reduce foodborne disease occur at the federal, state, and local levels. At the federal level, the USDA's Food Safety and Inspection Service (FSIS) is central. Notably, the USDA introduced the Pathogen Reduction and Hazard Analysis and Critical Control Point (HACCP) program in 1996, which provides more intensive surveillance of foodborne infections in 10 states to ensure the safety of the meat, poultry, and egg products supply. "The HACCP-Based Inspection Models Project was developed by the FSIS to produce a flexible, more efficient, fully integrated meat and poultry inspection system" (USDA, 2010).

PulseNet is another federal initiative to ensure safe food, a collaborative of the USDA/FSIS, FDA, and CDC. The objectives of the program are to detect foodborne disease case clusters by pulsed-field gel electrophoresis (PFGE) and facilitate early detection of outbreak sources (CDC, 2010e).

PulseNet is a national network of public health and food regulatory agency laboratories coordinated by the Centers for Disease Control and Prevention (CDC). The network consists of: state health departments, local health departments, and federal agencies (CDC, USDA/FSIS, FDA).

PulseNet participants perform standardized molecular subtyping (or "fingerprinting") of foodborne disease-causing bacteria by pulsed-field gel electrophoresis (PFGE). PFGE can be used to distinguish strains of organisms such as *Escherichia coli* O157:H7, *Salmonella*, *Shigella*, *Listeria*, or *Campylobacter* at the DNA level. DNA "fingerprints," or patterns, are submitted electronically to a dynamic database at the CDC. These databases are available on-demand to participants—this allows for rapid comparison of the patterns.

TABLE 4.2   Common Foodborne Disease Agents

Etiology	Incubation Period	Signs and Symptoms	Duration	Associated Foods	Laboratory Testing/Treatment
Bacillus cereus (preformed enterotoxin)	1–6 hours	Sudden onset of severe nausea and vomiting	24 hours	Improperly refrigerated cooked or fried rice, meats.	—Normally a clinical diagnosis; Send stool and food specimens to reference laboratory for culture and toxin. —Supportive care.
B. cereus (diarrheal toxin)	10–16 hours	Abdominal cramps, watery diarrhea, nausea.	24–48 hours	Meats, stews, gravies, vanilla sauce.	—Testing not necessary unless outbreak. —Supportive care.
Campylobacter jejuni	2–5 days	Diarrhea, cramps, fever, and vomiting; diarrhea may be bloody.	2–10 days	Raw and undercooked poultry, unpasteurized milk, contaminated water.	—Routine stool culture; requires special media. —Supportive care. For severe cases: erythromycin and quinolones.
Enterohemorrhagic Escherichia coli (EHEC) Including **E. coli O157:H7**	1–8 days	Severe diarrhea—often bloody, abdominal pain, vomiting. Rarely fever, more common in younger than 4 years of age.	5–10 days	Undercooked beef especially hamburger, unpasteurized milk and juice, raw fruits and vegetables (e.g., sprouts), salami (rarely), and contaminated water.	—Stool Culture; E. coli O157:H7 requires special media to grow. —Supportive care, monitor renal function, hemoglobin, and platelets. E. coli O157:H7 associated with hemolytic uremic syndrome (HUS). Antibiotics may promote HUS.

Organism	Incubation	Symptoms	Source	Diagnosis/Treatment
Enterotoxigenic E. coli (ETEC)	1–3 days	Watery diarrhea, abdominal cramps, some vomiting.	Water or food contaminated with human feces.	—Stool culture, ETEC requires special laboratory techniques. —Supportive care. Antibiotics (TMP-SMX and quinolones) are rarely needed except in severe cases.
Salmonella	6–72 hours	Diarrhea, fever, abdominal cramps, vomiting.	Contaminated eggs, poultry, unpasteurized milk or juice, cheese, contaminated raw fruits and vegetables (alfalfa sprouts, melons)	—Routine stool cultures. —Supportive care. Other than for *Salmonella* typhi, antibiotics are not indicated unless extra-intestinal spread. Consider ampicillin, gentamicin, TMP-SMX, or quinolones.
Shigella	24–48 hours	Abdominal cramps, fever, and diarrhea. Stools may contain blood and mucus.	Food or water contaminated with human fecal material. Usually person-to-person spread, fecal–oral transmission, raw vegetables, salads sandwiches.	—Routine stool cultures. —Supportive care. TMP-SMX recommended if susceptible; nalidixic acid or other quinolones if resistant.
Staphylococcus aureus (preformed enterotoxin)	1–6 hours	Sudden onset of severe nausea and vomiting. Possible diarrhea and fever. Abdominal cramps.	Unrefrigerated or improperly refrigerated meats, potato and egg salads, and cream pastries.	—Normally a clinical diagnosis. Stool, vomitus, and food can be tested for toxin and cultured if indicated. —Supportive care.

FoodNet is another federal program aimed at decreasing foodborne illness (CDC, 2010a):

> The Foodborne Diseases Active Surveillance Network (FoodNet) is the principal foodborne disease component of CDC's Emerging Infections Program (EIP). FoodNet is a collaborative project of the CDC, ten EIP sites, the U.S. Department of Agriculture (USDA), and the Food and Drug Administration (FDA).
>
> The project consists of active surveillance for foodborne diseases and related epidemiologic studies designed to help public health officials better understand the epidemiology of foodborne diseases in the United States. The objectives are:
>
> - Determine the burden of foodborne illness in the United States
> - Monitor trends in the burden of specific foodborne illness over time
> - Attribute the burden of foodborne illness to specific foods and settings
> - Disseminate information that can lead to improvements in public health practice and the development of interventions to reduce the burden of foodborne illness.

Most areas of the country have restaurant and food preparation inspection systems provided by state or local health departments. Because the most common factors responsible for foodborne disease outbreaks are improper holding temperature, poor hygiene of food handlers, contaminated equipment, and inadequate cooking, these efforts to inspect and maintain safe food preparation in local areas are vital.

Nationwide expansion and improvement of each of these programs would significantly improve the surveillance of documented foodborne diseases and reduce report and investigation time for each of these infections. Most individual cases of foodborne disease require approximately 2 weeks of time to investigate effectively, but with intensive active surveillance, that time can be reduced to 5–7 days. In addition, food irradiation has been endorsed by the WHO, CDC, FDA, USDA, and the American Medical Association. Currently, the European Commission's Food and Feed Safety section has approved food irradiation for certain purposes. Since 1997, the United States has irradiated fresh meat, and, in August of 2008, the FDA approved the irradiation of iceberg lettuce and spinach. In 2001, the CDC estimated that irradiation of these high-risk foods could prevent nearly 1 million cases of bacterial foodborne disease each year, 8,500 hospitalizations, more than 6,000 catastrophic illnesses, and 350 deaths in the United States. (Tauxe, 2001).

New initiatives would improve food safety, as well. These include more rapid and sensitive laboratory methods for detecting enteropathogens in food during processing and in random sampling of final products. In addition, commercial foods could be required to bar code, which would permit immediate tracing of a food item from a specific farm, plant, or distribution center. This would greatly accelerate the resolutions of foodborne outbreaks such as the *Salmonella* outbreaks traced to Mexican peppers. In addition, we could pursue new approaches to the feeding of poultry, swine, and cattle that can reduce the colonization by bacteria such as *E. coli*, *Salmonella*, and *Campylobacter*.

RISING PUBLIC HEALTH RISK OF UNVACCINATED CHILDREN

Childhood vaccinations are an essential public health strategy to maintaining a healthy population of children, adolescents, and adults free of infectious diseases. The CDC's ACIP provides a list of childhood vaccinations recommended for all children. By age 18, a child immunized according to schedule will have been vaccinated against (CDC, 2010f):

- Hepatitis B;
- Rotavirus;
- Diphtheria and tetanus toxoids and acellular pertussis;
- Haemophilus influenzae type b;
- Pneumococcal;
- Poliovirus;
- Influenza (seasonal);
- Measles, mumps, rubella;
- Varicella;
- Hepatitis A;
- Meningococcal; and
- Human papillomavirus.

The National Immunization Survey (NIS), sponsored by the National Center for Immunizations and Respiratory Diseases (NCIRD), monitors immunization coverage among children in the United States (CDC, 2010c). The results from the 2008 survey show that, overall, about 90% of children aged 19–35 months of all races and ethnicities are fully or partially immunized against the major childhood diseases: hepatitis B, diphtheria and tetanus toxoids and acellular pertussis, haemophilus influenzae type b, pneumococcal, poliovirus, measles, mumps, rubella, and varicella.

The percentage of children vaccinated, however, has been declining. In 1991, less than 1% of children were exempted from childhood vaccinations by states and localities. By 2004, nearly 2.5% of children were exempted. There are medical and religious exemptions in nearly all states. Personal exemptions, on the other hand, exist in 21 states, including California, Texas, Ohio, and Minnesota. They are not permitted in the states of New York, New Jersey, Florida, and Connecticut. This situation has led to more clusters of childhood diseases that were previously rare and is becoming an increasingly serious public health risk to many unvaccinated children and immunocompromised individuals of any age. Unvaccinated children are susceptible to serious illnesses, such as measles. In addition, they present a danger to others who may not be fully protected. Personal or philosophical exemptions are considered potentially dangerous and bad public health policy (Omer et al., 2006). Following is a commentary written by Paul Offit and published in the *Wall Street Journal* in 2007, discussing the problem of unvaccinated children.

Fatal Exemption: Relationship Between Vaccine Exemptions and Rates of Disease. Commentary by Paul Offit, MD, Director, Vaccine Education Center, Children's Hospital of Philadelphia. Published in *Wall Street Journal*, January 20, 2007.

Last month [October 2006] the *Journal of the American Medical Association* (JAMA) published a study that received little attention from the press and, as a consequence, the public. The study examined the incidence of whooping cough (pertussis) in children whose parents had chosen not to vaccinate them; the results were concerning.

Vaccines are recommended by the Centers for Disease Control and Prevention (CDC) and professional societies, such as the American Academy of Pediatrics. But these organizations can't enforce their recommendations; only states can do that—usually when children enter day care centers and elementary schools—in the form of mandates. State vaccine mandates have been on the books since the early 1900s; but aggressive enforcement of them didn't occur until much later, born from tragedy.

In 1963 the first measles vaccine was introduced in the United States. Measles is a highly contagious disease that can infect the lungs causing fatal pneumonia, or the brain causing encephalitis. Before the measles vaccine, measles caused 100,000 American children to be hospitalized and 3,000 to die every year. In the early 1970s, public health officials found that states with vaccine mandates had rates of measles that were 50 percent lower than states without mandates. As a consequence, all states worked toward requiring children to get vaccines. Now every state has some form of vaccine mandates.

But not all children are subject to these mandates. All fifty states have medical exemptions to vaccines, such as a serious allergy to a vaccine component. Forty-eight states also have religious exemptions; Amish groups, for example, traditionally reject vaccines, believing that clean living and a healthy diet are all that are needed to avoid vaccine-preventable diseases. And twenty states have philosophical exemptions; in some states these exemptions are easy to obtain, by simply signing your name at the bottom of a form; and in others they're much harder, requiring notarization, annual renewal, a signature from a local health official, or a personally written letter from a parent.

The JAMA study examined the relationship between vaccine exemptions and rates of disease. The authors found that between 1991 and 2004 the percentage of children whose parents had chosen to exempt them from vaccines increased by 6 percent per year, resulting in a 2.5-fold increase. This increase occurred almost solely in states where philosophical exemptions were easy to obtain. Worse, states with easy-to-obtain philosophical exemptions had twice as many children suffering from pertussis—a disease that causes inflammation of the windpipe and breathing tubes, pneumonia and, in about twenty infants every year, death—than states with hard-to-obtain philosophical exemptions.

The finding that lower immunization rates caused higher rates of disease shouldn't be surprising. In 1991 a massive epidemic of measles in Philadelphia centered on a group that chose not to immunize its children; as a consequence nine children died from measles. In the late 1990s, severe outbreaks of pertussis occurred in Colorado and Washington among children whose parents feared pertussis vaccine. And in 2005 a 17-year-old unvaccinated girl, unknowingly having brought measles back with her from Romania, attended a church gathering of 500 people in Indiana and caused the largest outbreak of measles in the United States in ten years; an outbreak that was limited to children whose parents had chosen not to vaccinate them. These events showed that for contagious diseases like measles and pertussis it's hard for unvaccinated children to successfully hide among herds of vaccinated children.

Some would argue that philosophical exemptions are a necessary pop-off valve for a society that requires children to be injected with biological agents for the common good. But as anti-vaccine activists continue to push more states to allow for easy philosophical exemptions one thing is clear, more and more children will suffer and occasionally die from vaccine preventable diseases.

When it comes to issues of public health and safety we invariably have laws. Many of these laws are strictly enforced and immutable. For example, we don't allow philosophical exemptions to restraining young children in car seats or smoking in restaurants or stopping at stop signs. And the notion of requiring vaccines for school entry, while it seems to tear at the very heart of a country founded on the basis of individual rights and freedoms, saves lives. Given the increasing number of states allowing philosophical exemptions to vaccines, at some point we are going to be forced to decide whether it is our inalienable right to catch and transmit potentially fatal infections.

Measles: A Case Study

Measles is still a worldwide health problem, and a global effort by the WHO and the United Nations Children's Emergency Fund (UNICEF) to control measles is underway, with some reduction in cases:

Because of limited disease surveillance and death registration in many countries with weak infrastructure and high measles burden, current routine reporting systems are inadequate for monitoring global measles mortality. Different modeling approaches have been used to estimate the global number of measles deaths. Published estimates from these approaches vary both in level and precision and have wide uncertainty bounds that overlap. A panel of six experts was convened in January 2005 to advise WHO on how best to monitor progress toward the 2005 measles mortality reduction goal. The panel noted strengths and weaknesses in various approaches to estimating measles mortality but endorsed the use of surveillance data (where they are reliable) and a natural history model (where surveillance data are unreliable) because the latter accounts for recent changes in vaccination coverage and is therefore better suited for monitoring trends. However, the panel recommended that uncertainty bounds around the point estimates be calculated to indicate the lack of precision.

On the basis of results from the natural history model, overall global measles mortality decreased 39%, from 873,000 deaths (uncertainty bounds: 645,000—1,196,000 deaths) in 1999 to 530,000 deaths (bounds: 383,000—731,000 deaths) in 2003. The largest reduction was in Africa, where estimated measles mortality decreased by 46% during this period. (CDC, 2005).

As of 2000, measles is no longer considered endemic in the United States, and all cases of measles reported are believed to be related directly or secondarily to international importation. Because measles continues to be endemic throughout the world, the CDC recommends full measles immunity for any individual traveling outside the country. Recent large outbreaks have been reported in Great Britain, Switzerland, Austria, Italy, and Israel. Cases have been identified throughout Europe and also in Central Asia and Japan.

New York reported a confirmed measles case in an unvaccinated 13-year-old child within the last five years. The child traveled to Italy from July 1 to July 20, which included a brief stop in Switzerland from July 2 to July 3. Beginning the night of July 24, the child exhibited upper respiratory symptoms, was seen by her provider on July 25 and prescribed Zithromax (azithromycin), which she completed on July 30. On July 29, she developed a cough and coryza and visited an area shopping mall. On August 1, she was again seen by her provider with symptoms of coryza, runny eyes, rash, and fever of 103°F. Antibiotics were prescribed for a diagnosis of pharyngitis and otitis media. On August 2, she was seen at a local emergency department with reported fever higher than 101°F for 4 days; cough; red, watery eyes; runny nose; and a nonpruritic rash that developed on August 1 from face to body. The emergency department provider described the rash as erythematous, macular, and papular. On August 4, a serology for measles was drawn at another provider office. Preliminary serology results were received by the county health department on August 14. Both the measles IgM and IgG were positive and interpreted as indicating current or recent disease. The serum sample was immediately sent to Wadsworth Diagnostic Immunology Laboratory where the measles disease was confirmed on August 15.

The county health department responded immediately to the preliminary laboratory results received on August 14 and started a thorough case and contact investigation. Following the confirmed results, notices of exposure were completed to all: family physicians, pediatricians, infectious disease specialists, emergency department physicians, and other health care providers in the county. The notice stated the following:

> The York State Department of Health had a confirmed serology for measles in a 13 year old who had not been immunized. The typical measles rash began on August 1, with coryza and conjunctivitis beginning several days before. The period of communicability was calculated as beginning 5 days before onset of the rash and continuing 5 days after. People who were not immune and who had contact with the child from July 27 through August 6 were considered exposed to measles. Measles is highly infectious by droplet spread, or by direct contact with secretions from the nose or throat or from soiled articles. People who come into a room - an exam or waiting room - for up to two hours after an infected person are also considered exposed. In addition to her normal activities, the child visited the local mall on July 29, within the period of communicability. Non-immune persons exposed may develop measles for up to 18 days after contact. Measures that can be taken after discovery of exposure include administration of the measles/mumps/rubella (MMR) vaccination; this can be effective if done within 72 hours of exposure. Immuneglobulin is also effective if given within 6 days of exposure. In this particular case, we are now outside the window. Department of Health Communicable Disease personnel are asking physicians and providers to be aware of this case of measles and to be alert for signs and symptoms of this disease in non-immune patients. Clinical presentation with serology is key to diagnosis. Any positive serology should be confirmed by the State Laboratory. County public health staff is available to assist with any questions. Due to the delay in notification, susceptible contacts are not eligible for post exposure prophylaxis. They are being individually notified of the symptoms of measles and asked to seek medical care after notifying their provider of symptoms.

This case ended without further development of measles in the unvaccinated population, and the child recovered fully. However, the risk of a measles outbreak was a serious threat to the unvaccinated.

Immunization Successes

The long-term benefits of wide-scale immunizations of children are clear, as noted in the following graphs (see Figures 4.2–4.8):

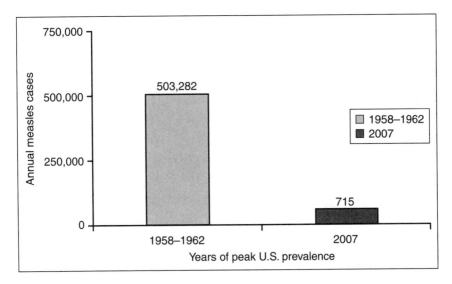

FIGURE 4.2   Impact of Vaccinations on Measles in U.S. from the NIH, National Institute of Allergy and Infectious Diseases. Adapted by David G. Graham, MD, Suffolk County, New York, 2009.

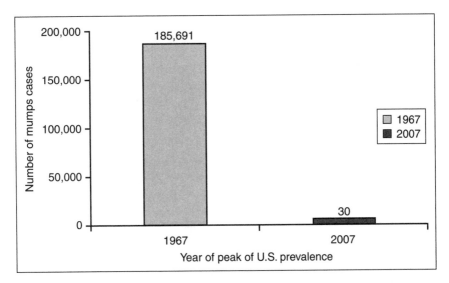

FIGURE 4.3   Impact of Vaccinations on Mumps in U.S. from the NIH, National Institute of Allergy and Infectious Diseases. Adapted by David G. Graham, MD, Suffolk County, New York, 2009.

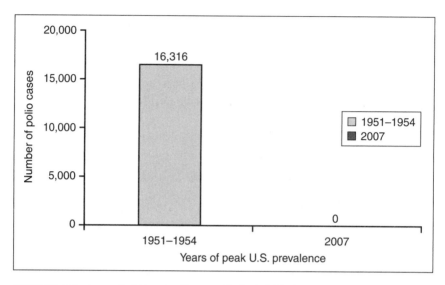

FIGURE 4.4   Impact of Vaccinations on Polio in U.S. from the NIH, National Institute of Allergy and Infectious Diseases. Adapted by David G. Graham, MD, Suffolk County, New York, 2009.

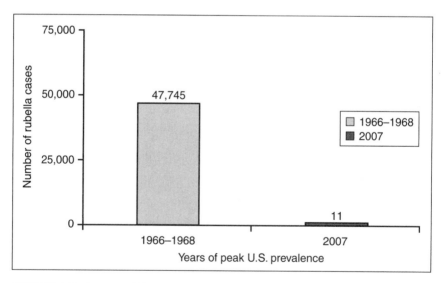

FIGURE 4.5   Impact of Vaccinations on Rubella in U.S. from the NIH, National Institute of Allergy and Infectious Diseases. Adapted by David G. Graham, MD, Suffolk County, New York, 2009.

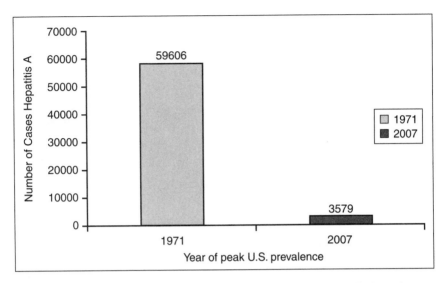

FIGURE 4.6   Impact of Vaccinations on Hepatitis A Disease in U.S. from the NIH, National Institute of Allergy and Infectious Diseases. Adapted by David G. Graham, MD, Suffolk County, New York, 2009.

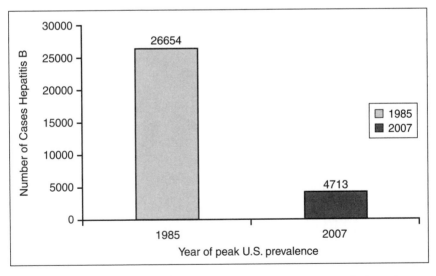

FIGURE 4.7   Impact of Vaccinations on Hepatitis B Disease in U.S. from the NIH, National Institute of Allergy and Infectious Diseases. Adapted by David G. Graham, MD, Suffolk County, New York, 2009.

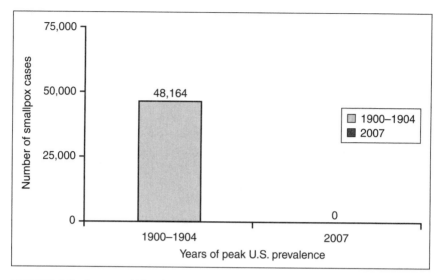

FIGURE 4.8   Impact of Vaccinations on Smallpox in U.S. from the NIH, National Institute of Allergy and Infectious Diseases. Adapted by David G. Graham, MD, Suffolk County, New York, 2009.

INVESTIGATION OF A DISEASE OUTBREAK OR EPIDEMIC

There are several fundamental steps necessary to conduct an investigation of an infectious disease outbreak. They are:

- Verify the diagnosis of the disease that is suspect or under investigation;
- Establish the existence of an outbreak of disease or an epidemic;
- Characterize the distribution of disease cases by the variables of person, place, and time;
- Develop a hypothesis that can explain the observed distribution of cases; and
- Institute control measures as early as possible.

Verify Diagnosis

To verify the diagnosis of an outbreak of disease, the epidemiologist considers several factors.

- Laboratory tests may be used in a diagnosis of the disease. The investigator must make certain that the results are reliable by having the test confirmed by a trustworthy laboratory or repeated by another laboratory to confirm the original diagnosis. In each state, there is a diagnostic laboratory that is approved for this purpose.

■ Use clinical criteria when the laboratory results are not entirely reliable or may not be available in a timely fashion. Some illnesses may be very mild or not apparent in laboratory tests. Similarly, there may be other unrelated illnesses that may be part of the initial count of cases in the outbreak investigation.

■ Epidemiologic criteria may be added to the laboratory information and to the clinical criteria to further restrict the number of cases that are under investigation. For example, during the 1976 investigation of Legionnaires' disease in Philadelphia, there was no laboratory test available to confirm the clinical suspicion of the illness. Consequently, a clinical diagnosis of a respiratory illness with a fever was created. Because the clinical definition of a febrile respiratory illness was so broad as to include a very large number of unrelated cases, an additional component in the epidemiologic investigation was added to the case definition: an individual needed to have specific clinical findings and also to have attended the American Legion Convention in Philadelphia or entered one of the hotels where the convention itself was held during a specific period. This additional information helped restrict the suspect cases to determine and make a more accurate count of cases.

Establish Existence of Outbreak

If an outbreak or an epidemic is considered an unusual occurrence of the disease in a defined population during a specific period, it must be documented. It could be a common disease in an unusual segment of the population (e.g., pneumonia in persons who attended the 1976 American Legion Convention in Philadelphia) or an unusual disease in a common segment of the population (e.g., the occurrence of a specific form of pneumonia caused by *Pneumocystis carinii* in young homosexual men), which was seen as a common factor in HIV-infected individuals in the early days of AIDS epidemic in the 1980s. When trying to establish the existence of an outbreak of disease or an epidemic, epidemiologists do the following:

■ Identify unreported or unrecognized cases that may be part of the specific outbreak of disease. These additional cases may be found by surveying hospitals, laboratories, physicians, and family and friends of the known cases.

■ Determine the population at risk for developing the disease in question. This may be a specific classroom of children, or the entire school, or a much larger community of people.

■ Compare the incidence of new cases of the disease in the population now, with the previous period, using the case count as a numerator and the population at risk as the denominator. Take into consideration seasonal variations, while comparing the incidence of new cases with the same period in previous years.

Characterize Distribution of Cases by Person, Place, and Time

Understanding the cause of an outbreak results from the proper analysis of the distribution of cases by time, place, and person.

Time

The variable time is used to begin the construction of an epidemic curve, which is a graph showing the distribution of cases (on the Y-axis) by the date of onset of the illness in hours, days, weeks, or months (on the X-axis). The shape of this curve may suggest either a common source outbreak or person-to-person transmission. A point source of exposure is suggested if all cases occur within one incubation period of the disease (i.e., the time in which the disease was incubating before signs and symptoms of disease occurred). Common source outbreaks of disease result from the exposure of individuals to the same causal factor or pathogen(s) including contaminated water, milk, food, or in other ingested, consumed, inhaled, or absorbed substances. Exposure to a contaminated source may be temporary or continuous. In the case of instantaneous or temporary contamination, transmission occurs in the following fashion (see Figure 4.9):

One characteristic feature of a temporary or instantaneous common source epidemic (sometimes called *point source*) is that all cases occur during a period that covers the range of one incubation period (see Figure 4.10). This pattern can be observed only if secondary cases do not result from the primary case.

Common source outbreaks differ from contact, or progressive, outbreaks whereby infection is transmitted from a patient or a carrier to one or more susceptibles, characterized by the following epidemic curve (see Figure 4.11).

The shape of the epidemic curve in contact or progressive outbreak depends on the infectivity of the pathogen, its ability to survive outside of human host, the proportion of susceptibles in the community, and the length of the carrier state.

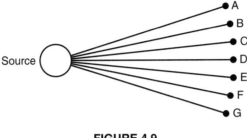

FIGURE 4.9

Cases that occur over several different incubation periods suggest either person-to-person transmission or a continuing common source of exposure and outbreak. If the incubation period of the disease is known, the curve indicates the probable time and possible source of the infection. If the time of exposure can be determined, the incubation period of the disease can be identified.

If the time of exposure is known, the incubation period can be used to establish a diagnosis in a foodborne disease outbreak. For example, if there is a chemical food poisoning due to the ingestion of copper, the incubation period can be measured in minutes. Staphylococcal food poisoning has an onset in 1–6 hours. Other foodborne bacteria that cause disease outbreaks are *Bacillus cereus*, with an incubation period of 10–16 hours; *Salmonella*, with an incubation period of 6–72 hours; and *Shigella*, with an incubation period of 24–48 hours.

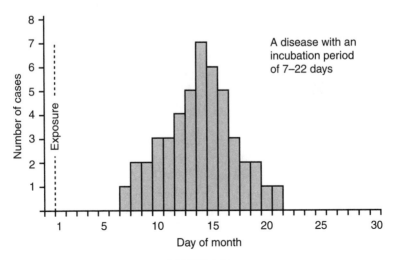

FIGURE 4.10

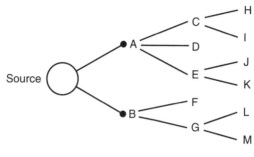

FIGURE 4.11

Place

The variable place can be used to detect a source of infection by identification of spatial clustering of cases. Cases can be plotted by the place where the individuals reside, work, or attend school, or by any other geographic location. Because clustering of cases may only reflect population density, maps should be drawn comparing the rates of outbreak in different geographic areas.

Person

The variable person can be used to compare the characteristics of the population contracting the disease to the characteristics of the population without the disease.

Develop and Test Hypothesis

In developing a hypothesis, the unusual or odd case may be extremely helpful. The exceptions frequently provide important information and may help explain the source of an infection, the mode of disease transmission, or the normal background of the disease. The following procedure is standard:

- Demonstrate the differences in the attack rates of people who were exposed and not exposed to the source of infection. The cases must be shown to be exposed more often to the risk factor than the group of individuals, known as the *controls*, who are not ill.
- Apply statistical tests to the data to indicate statistical differences between cases and controls.
- Collect clinical and environmental specimens if they are available for processing in an appropriate laboratory.

■ If the laboratory data does not support the epidemiologic data, ignore the laboratory data.

Formulate a conclusion based on all pertinent evidence and the results of the hypothesis testing.
A final report describing all aspects of the investigation should be prepared.

Institute Control Measures

Institute control measures as early as possible in the outbreak investigation to prevent further occurrence of illness. Control or intervention measures are directed at one of the conditions or events in the infectious disease process. The control measures selected depend on the disease under consideration. For example, if a contaminated food is a suspected source of the infection, remove that food and submit to testing.

Two Investigations of *Salmonella* Outbreaks

In 2008, two nationwide outbreaks of *Salmonella* infection occurred. Between April and August 2008, *Salmonella* Saintpaul enteritis was diagnosed in more than 1,400 people in 43 states, the District of Columbia, and Canada. Ultimately, 282 people were hospitalized and two elderly patients died from the *Salmonella* infection. In the initial investigation by the state health departments and the CDC (Maki, 2009), the source of contamination was thought to be tomatoes grown in the southwestern United States, although this was never proved by laboratory findings. Because of those initial investigations and adverse publicity, tomato consumption in the United States dropped dramatically and the industry lost hundreds of millions of dollars. After several months of further investigation, the outbreak of *Salmonella* was isolated from jalapeño and serrano peppers that had been grown on one Mexican farm. The CDC concluded that the outbreak of *Salmonella* derived from contaminated peppers that were eaten raw and may have accompanied tomatoes, which could have explained the misleading results from the early investigation (CDC, 2009a).

In a second *Salmonella* outbreak, which began in September 2008 and continued into 2009, *Salmonella typhimurium* enteritis was diagnosed in more than 600 people in 44 states and in Canada by February 2009. The CDC traced the outbreak to contamination of one peanut butter producer in Georgia and other manufacturers that used the contaminated peanut butter. More than half the cases were children and hundreds of patients were hospitalized. The outbreak may have contributed to eight deaths. Because of this outbreak, there was a recall of all peanut butter products produced by the company since early 2008, which involved more than 400 food products including cookies, crackers, cereal, candy, ice cream, and pet foods. The investigation revealed that *Salmonella* had been isolated from the company's peanut butter or peanut paste during internal quality control efforts on at least a dozen occasions in the previous year, but no action had been taken to end the contamination. The company is now under criminal investigation (CDC, 2009b). It has been estimated that in outbreaks of *Salmonella*, for every case that is identified by clinical laboratory tests and culture, there are approximately 38 additional undetected cases, meaning that each of these two outbreaks may have affected more than 20,000 persons.

REFERENCES

Belshe, R. B. (2005). The origins of pandemic influenza—Lessons from the 1918 virus. *New England Journal of Medicine, 353*(21), 2209–2211.

Centers for Disease Control and Prevention.(2004). Diagnosis and management of foodborne illnesses: A primer for physicians and other health care professionals. *Morbidity and Mortality Weekly Report, 53*(RR-4), 1–33.

Centers for Disease Control and Prevention. (2005). Progress in reducing measles mortality–Worldwide, 1999–2003. *Morbidity and Mortality Weekly Report, 54*(8), 200–203.

Centers for Disease Control and Prevention. (2006a). New laboratory assay for diagnostic testing of avian influenza A/H5 (Asian Lineage). *Morbidity and Mortality Weekly Report, 55*(Early Release), 1.

Centers for Disease Control and Prevention. (2006b). High levels of adamantane resistance among influenza A (H3N2) viruses and interim guidelines for use of antiviral agents—United States, 2005–2006 influenza season. *Morbidity and Mortality Weekly Report, 55*(2), 44–46.

Centers for Disease Control and Prevention. (2009a). *Investigation of outbreak of infections caused by Salmonella Saintpaul*. Retrieved February 11, 2009 from http://www.cdc.gov/salmonella/saintpaul/jalapeno/

Centers for Disease Control and Prevention. (2009b). *Investigation update: Outbreak of Salmonella typhimurium infections, 2008–2009*. Retrieved October 20, 2010, from http://www.cdc.gov/salmonella/typhimurium/update.html

Centers for Disease Control and Prevention. (2009c). *Epidemiology and prevention of vaccine-preventable diseases* (11th ed.). Washington, DC: Public Health Foundation.

Centers for Disease Control and Prevention. (2010a). *FoodNet*. Retrieved July 15, 2010, from http://www.cdc.gov/foodnet/.

Centers for Disease Control and Prevention. (2010b). *Hepatitis B information for health professionals.* Retrieved June 22, 2010, from http://www.cdc.gov/hepatitis/HBV/PerinatalXmtn.htm

Centers for Disease Control and Prevention. (2010c). *National immunization survey.* Retrieved July 22, 2010, from http://www.cdc.gov/nis/

Centers for Disease Control and Prevention. (2010d). *National notifiable diseases surveillance system.* Retrieved July 19, 2010, from http://www.cdc.gov/ncphi/disss/nndss/nndsshis.htm

Centers for Disease Control and Prevention. (2010e). *PulseNet.* Retrieved July 15, 2010, from http://www.cdc.gov/pulsenet/

Centers for Disease Control and Prevention. (2010f). Recommended immunization schedules for persons aged 0 through 18 years–United States, 2010. *Morbidity and Mortality Weekly Report, 58*(5,152), 1–4.

Centers for Disease Control and Prevention. (2010g). *Viral hepatitis—funded partners: Perinatal hepatitis B prevention coordinators.* Retrieved June 22, 2010 from http://www.cdc.gov/hepatitis/Partners/PeriHepBCoord.htm

Hayden, F. G. (2006). Antiviral resistance in influenza viruses—implications for management and pandemic response. *New England Journal of Medicine, 354*(8), 785–788.

Maki, D. G. (2006). Don't eat the spinach–Controlling foodborne infectious disease. *New England Journal of Medicine, 355*(19), 1952–1955.

Maki, D. G. (2009). Coming to grips with foodborne infection—Peanut butter, peppers, and nationwide salmonella outbreaks. *New England Journal of Medicine, 360*, 949–953.

Moore, P. (2007). *The little book of pandemics.* London: Elwin Street Limited.

Occupational Safety and Health Administration, U.S. Department of Labor. (2010). *Foodborne disease: Control and prevention.* Retrieved July 5, 2010, from http://www.osha.gov/SLTC/foodbornedisease/control.html

Omer, S. B., Pan, W. K. Y., Halsey, N. A., Stokley, S., Moulton, L. H., Navar, A. M., et al. (2006). Nonmedical exemptions to school immunization requirements: Secular trends and association of state policies with pertussis incidence. *Journal of American Medical Association, 296*, 1757–1763.

Taubenberger, J. K., Reid, A. H., Lourens, R. M., Wang, R., Jin, G., & Fanning, T. G. (2005). Characterization of the 1918 influenza virus polymerase genes. *Nature, 437*, 889–893.

Tauxe, R. V. (2001). Food safety and irradiation: Protecting the public from foodborne infections. *Emerging Infectious Diseases, 7*(Suppl.), 516–521.

Tumpey, T. M., Basler, C. F., Aguilar, P. V., Zeng, H., Solórzano, A., Swayne, D. E., et al. (2005). Characterization of the reconstructed 1918 Spanish influenza pandemic virus. *Science, 310*, 77–80.

Ungchusak, K., Auewarakul, P., Dowell, S. F., Kitphati, R., Auwanit, W., Puthavathana, P., et al. (2005). Probable person-to-person transmission of avian influenza A (H5N1). *New England Journal of Medicine, 352*, 333–340.

United States Department of Agriculture, Food Safety and Inspection Service. (2010). *HACCP and pathogen reduction*. Retrieved July 15, 2010, from http://www.fsis.usda.gov/Science/hazard_analysis_&_pathogen_reduction/
World Health Organization. (2010). *WHO Global Influenza Surveillance Network*. Retrieved July 15, 2010, from http://www.who.int/csr/disease/influenza/surveillance/en/

Note:

We wish to acknowledge Mahfouz H. Zaki, MD, MPH, DrPH, formerly distinguished university professor of Preventive Medicine and Public Health at Downstate Medical Center in Brooklyn and adjunct professor of Preventive Medicine at State University of New York at Stony Brook, for his contributions to this section. Sadly, Dr. Zaki passed away in 2009.

5

Injuries and Noninfectious Diseases

INTRODUCTION

Infectious disease control has historical significance for public health—having provided many, if not most of, public health's early successes—and it remains a major component of public health practice today, as discussed in the previous chapter. However, the scope of public health in the United States has steadily increased since the 19th century in response to changes in the health problems that have the greatest impact on morbidity and mortality. Today, the 10 leading causes of death, overall, in the United States are diseases of the heart, malignant neoplasms, cerebrovascular diseases, chronic lower respiratory diseases, unintentional injuries, diabetes mellitus, Alzheimer's disease, influenza and pneumonia, nephritis, nephritic syndrome and nephrosis, and septicemia. Although the order is different, these are the same 10 causes of death for men and women, with the exception that suicide is a leading cause of death for men and not women, and septicemia for women and not men. The list of 10 leading causes of death remains much the same for different race and ethnic groups, as well. The most notable differences are for males: (a) homicide is a leading cause of death for Black men, but not White or Hispanic men; (b) suicide is a leading cause of death among White and Hispanic men, but not Black men; (c) HIV is a leading cause for Black men, but not White and Hispanic males; (d) Alzheimer's disease and pneumonia and influenza are leading causes among White men, but not Hispanic and Black males; (e) conditions originating in the perinatal period are a leading cause of death for Black and Hispanic men, but not White males (National Center for Health Statistics [NCHS], 2010b, Table 28). Only 2 on the list of the 10 leading causes of death—pneumonia and influenza and septicemia—are infectious diseases. Because of their predominant effect on mortality and morbidity, injuries and noninfectious diseases have assumed a public health importance equal to infectious diseases.

The number of problems tackled within the area of injury prevention and noninfectious disease control is tremendous. Following is a partial overview of the Centers for Disease Control and Prevention (CDC) agenda, which establishes and reflects the public health agenda for the nation. The list gives an indication of the scope, variety, and number of issues related to injuries and noninfectious diseases that are targeted by public health (CDC, 2010d).

- Diseases and conditions:
  ADHD, birth defects, cancer, diabetes, fetal alcohol syndrome . . .
- Emergency preparedness and response:
  bioterrorism, chemical and radiation emergencies, severe weather . . .
- Environmental health:
  air pollution, carbon monoxide, lead, mold, water quality, climate change . . .
- Healthy living:
  bone health, physical activity, genetics, smoking prevention . . .
- Injury, violence and safety:
  brain injury, child abuse, falls, fires, poisoning, suicide, youth violence . . .
- Workplace safety and health:
  asbestos, chemical safety, construction, mining, office environments, respirators . . .

As a result of the range of issues related to injury prevention and noninfectious disease control, public health's response to each will not be discussed. Instead, we examine several childhood health problems that illustrate public health practice today in the areas of injury prevention and noninfectious disease control: (a) motor vehicle injuries among children; and (b) childhood obesity. Clearly unintentional injuries are a major problem, as they are a leading cause of death for males and females and among persons of the major race/ethnic groups. Obesity is a health behavior that contributes heavily to both cardiovascular disease and diabetes, both of which are on the top 10 causes of death for all groups.

Public health practice can be classified in the following way, and each practice example will be described using these categories:

Surveillance and Research
- Provide information on incidence, prevalence, and risk factors
- Conduct research on causes and consequences of health problem
- Evaluate effectiveness of interventions aimed at preventing and controlling health problem
- Develop data systems necessary for surveillance and research

Interventions to Prevent and Control Health Problem

■ Educate population at risk and related persons on how to reduce risk of health problem

■ Provide services for victims of health problem, including screening, treatment, and supportive services

■ Change social and/or physical environments to prevent health problems from occurring, which includes advocacy and policy solutions

We focus on the CDC activities, because these are usually the most comprehensive, and they often lead the state and local public heath efforts intellectually and through provision of technical and financial resources such as the cooperative agreements and block and categorical grants. However, we discuss state and local interventions, as this is the level where they are implemented.

MOTOR VEHICLE INJURIES

Unintentional injuries are a leading cause of death in the United States among all age, race, and ethnic groups, and motor vehicle accidents are the foremost cause of unintentional injuries. Motor vehicle accidents are also a leading cause of years of potential life lost before age 75 (NCHS, 2010b, Table 27). In addition, they are a leading cause of morbidity. Motor vehicle injuries are responsible for a major portion of all disabilities, which affect about 25% of all persons 18–64 years old and about 61% of persons 65 and over (NCHS, 2010b, Table 55).

The National Center for Injury Prevention and Control (CDC, 2010a), the CDC's lead division for injury prevention, reports the following statistics about the prevalence and cost, monetary and nonmonetary, of motor vehicle accidents:

■ In the United States, motor vehicle–related injuries are the leading cause of death among people ages 1–34, and nearly 4 million people sustain injuries that require an emergency department visit each year.

■ The economic impact of motor vehicle–related injuries is significant, with costs reaching approximately $230 billion in the United States in 2000.

■ Motor vehicle crashes prevent young people from achieving their full potential. Crashes are the leading cause of death for U.S. teens, accounting for more than one in three deaths in this age group. In 2008, on average, 11 teens ages 16–19 died every day from motor vehicle–related injuries.

■ In 2008, 968 children ages 14 years and younger died as occupants in crashes, and approximately 168,000 were injured.

■ Every day, on average, 32 people in the United States die in motor vehicle crashes that involve alcohol-impaired drivers. This amounts to one death every 45 minutes" (2010a, para. 3).

Not surprisingly, then, prevention of motor vehicle injuries and fatalities is a major public activity. The following description of public health practice related to prevention of motor vehicle accidents is taken mainly from the CDC (CDC, 2010e), which is the predominant actor in terms of agenda setting, surveillance and research, and source of funding. The emphasis is on childhood motor vehicle accidents.

Surveillance and Research

NCIPC conducts surveillance for all injuries, including motor vehicle, through the Public Health Injury Surveillance and Prevention Program (PHISP), which addresses injury and its variation by weather, geography, and population from state to state. PHISP (formally known as the Core State Injury Program) funds "core" capacity building and surveillance activities to prevent and control injuries—including traumatic brain injury (TBI). Currently, 30 states are funded to conduct basic surveillance (Part A). Some states are funded for Parts B, C, and D: Traumatic Brain Injury Extended Surveillance Program; Traumatic Brain Injury Emergency Department Surveillance Program; and Traumatic Brain Injury Service Linkage Program, respectively. The PHISP Program has three primary objectives:

■ Build a solid infrastructure for injury prevention and control;
■ Collect, analyze, and use injury data; and
■ Implement and evaluate interventions" (2010i, para. 2).

Fatal injury data are death certificate data from the *National Vital Statistics System*—deaths, death rates, and years of potential life lost (a measure of premature death) by specific causes of injury mortality and common causes of death. National estimates of injuries treated in U.S. hospital emergency departments are from the National Electronic Injury Surveillance System—All Injury Program (NEISS-AIP)—nonfatal injuries and nonfatal injury rates. Violent death data are from the National Violent

Death Reporting System (NVDRS)—violent incidents and deaths, death rates, and causes of injury mortality. These data are provided for 16 states only and are not nationally representative. Data are made available in WISQARS™ (Web-based Injury Statistics Query and Reporting System), an interactive database system that provides customized reports of injury-related data.

Recent activities and accomplishments of the PHISP include abstracting supplemental data on traumatic brain injuries from medical records to include information about alcohol use, severity of acute injury, and use of protective equipment such as automobile safety belts and child safety seats; conducting exploratory, emergency department-based surveillance to identify cases of mild traumatic brain injury; link individuals with services in their community; and helping states build capacity and strengthen essential infrastructure. "Most CDC-funded states use advisory committees to develop and prioritize injury plans. CDC encourages states to build coalitions with partners from academic, nonprofit, private, local government, and professional organizations. As a result, injury is widely recognized as a critical public health problem" (CDC, 2010i, para. 6).

Two surveillance and research initiatives aimed at reducing motor vehicle injuries among children are *Child Passenger Safety* and *Teen Drivers*. We will discuss the surveillance and research of both initiatives.

Child Passenger Safety

The Child Passenger Safety initiative focuses on increasing use of car and booster seats and seat belts; reducing impaired driving; and helping groups at risk including child passengers, teen drivers, and older adult drivers. There is also an interest in preventing pedestrian and bicycle injuries. The mission of the initiative is "to provide public health leadership to keep people safe on the road—every day; and to focus our research and programs on preventing injuries and deaths by increasing child safety seat and seat belt use, reducing alcohol-impaired driving, and helping groups at special risk: child passengers, teens, and American Indians/Alaska Natives" (CDC, 2010a, para. 7). Numerous studies have been conducted by the Child Passenger Safety initiative to understand the factors related to use of child safety restraints in motor vehicles and the risk of not using them (CDC, 2010b). See Table 5.1 for a summary of recent studies and their findings.

TABLE 5.1   CDC Research Activities Related to Child Passenger Safety, 2010

Child Counseling Study	Study: Cross-sectional telephone survey of randomly selected children in English or Spanish-speaking households in all 50 states and the District of Columbia. Main outcome measures: Respondent or their child received injury-prevention counseling from child's health care provider in the 12 months preceding the interview. Findings: Pediatric injury-prevention counseling, although not pervasive, was associated with safer behaviors among children, including use of bicycle helmets while biking and use of car seats and seat belts while riding in motor vehicles.
Modes of Travel to School	Study: Cross-sectional, nationally representative telephone survey among English and Spanish-speaking adults with at least one child between 5 and 14 years old in household. Main outcome measure: Mode of travel to school. Findings: Most common mode of travel to school was the family car (46.3%), followed by school bus (39.6%), and walking (14%). Among those who did not usually walk to school, distance (70.7%) was the most common barrier, followed by traffic danger (9.2%). Children in the South were less likely to walk to school than children in other regions (Northeast, North Central, and West). Distance to school was more commonly cited as a barrier to walking for older children than younger children. Efforts to promote walking to school may achieve better near-term success if focused on students who already live close to school.
Children's Hospital of Philadelphia Study	Study: Interview with parents of children younger than 16 years involved in a motor vehicle crash. Main outcome measures: Typical use of child restraints, type of restraint in use at the time of the crash, parent's understanding of child restraint laws in their state, and parent's understanding of how the motor vehicle crash had affected the child's daily life. Findings: Children had one or more physical limitations after the crash accounts for 3.3%. Parents were more likely to report physical limitations among older children (7.6%) than younger children (1%). Children with whiplash injuries were reported to have physical limitations after their injury accounts for 47%. Children who were not restrained optimally were nearly twice as likely as optimally restrained children to have physical limitations.
Alcohol-Impaired Driving and Children in the Household	Study: Second Injury Control and Risk Survey, a nationally representative cross-sectional telephone survey of adults. Main outcome measure: Alcohol-impaired driving by an adult with a child in the household Findings: An estimated 2.5 million adult drivers with children living in their households reported that they had been a recent alcohol-impaired driver.

Source: CDC, 2010b, para. 5–10.

The risk factors for motor vehicle injuries among children have been identified through the surveillance and research functions of the NCIPC. They include the following:

A Drinking Driver
- The rate of serious and fatal injuries to children can be reduced by half by using age- and size-appropriate car and booster seats.
- Fifteen percent of motor vehicle–related deaths among children ages 0–14 years involved a drinking driver.
- More than two thirds of motor vehicle–related deaths are among children riding with a drinking driver.

Improper or No Use of Seatbelt or Booster Seat
- Restraint use among young children often depends on the driver's seat belt use. Almost 40% of children riding with unbelted drivers were themselves unrestrained.
- Child restraint systems are often used incorrectly. One study found that 72% of nearly 3,500 observed car and booster seats were misused in a way that could be expected to increase a child's risk of injury during a crash.

Placing Child in the Front Seat of a Motor Vehicle
- Riding in the back seat reduces the risk of serious injury to children under 16 by 40%.

Teen Drivers

The risk factors for motor vehicle fatalities and injuries by teen drivers have been identified through the surveillance and research functions of the NCIPC (CDC, 2010h). They include the following:

Being 16–19 Years Old
- The risk of motor vehicle crashes is higher among 16- to 19-year-olds than among any other age group. In fact, per mile driven, teen drivers ages 16–19 are four times more likely than older drivers to crash.

Male Teen
- In 2006, the motor vehicle death rate for male drivers and passengers ages 15–19 was almost two times that of their female counterparts.

Teen Driving with Teen Passengers
- The presence of teen passengers increases the crash risk of unsupervised teen drivers. This risk increases with the number of teen passengers.

■ The presence of male teenage passengers increases the likelihood of risky driving behavior.

Newly Licensed Teen
■ Crash risk is particularly high during the first year that teenagers are eligible to drive.

Unsafe Driving Patterns
■ Teens are more likely than older drivers to underestimate dangerous situations and to be unable to recognize hazardous situations.
■ Teens are more likely than older drivers to speed and allow shorter headways (the distance from the front of one vehicle to the front of the next).

Failure to Wear Seatbelts
■ Teens have the lowest rate of seat belt use. In 2005, 10% of high school students reported they rarely or never wear seat belts when riding with someone else.
■ Male high school students (12.5%) were more likely than female students (7.8%) to rarely or never wear seat belts.
■ African American students (12%) and Hispanic students (13%) are more likely than White students (10.1%) to rarely or never wear seat belts.

Drinking and Driving
■ At all levels of blood alcohol concentration (BAC), the risk of involvement in a motor vehicle crash is greater for teens than older drivers.
■ In 2008, 25% of drivers ages 15–20 who died in motor vehicle crashes had a BAC of 0.08 g/dl or higher.
■ In a national survey conducted in 2007, nearly three out of ten teens reported that, within the previous month, they had ridden with a driver who had been drinking alcohol. One in ten reported having driven after drinking alcohol within the same 1-month period.
■ In 2008, nearly three out of every four teen drivers killed in motor vehicle crashes after drinking and driving were not wearing a seat belt.
■ In 2008, half of teen deaths from motor vehicle crashes occurred between 3 p.m. and midnight and 56% occurred on Friday, Saturday, or Sunday.
■ Thirty-seven percent of male drivers between 15 and 20 years old who were involved in fatal crashes in 2005 were speeding at the time of the crash and 26% had been drinking.

Interventions

As with most public health interventions, those for the *Child Passenger Safety* and *Teen Driver* initiatives are implemented at the state and local levels, so as to ensure culturally appropriate communications and in other ways be responsive to local needs, preferences, and conditions. In terms of primary and secondary prevention, interventions can be grouped as follows:

Primary Prevention
■ Educating population at risk and related persons on how to reduce risk of health problem.
■ Changing the social and/or physical environment to prevent health problems from occurring, including advocacy and policy solutions.

Secondary and Tertiary Prevention
■ Providing services for victims of health problem, including screening, treatment, and supportive services.

As we will see, both the *Child Passenger Safety* and *Teen Drivers* initiatives emphasize primary prevention, particularly education. This does not mean that providing health care services, that is, secondary and tertiary prevention, does not occur at other levels—state and local—for children who have sustained motor vehicle injuries. Much of this care—including screening, diagnosis, and treatment of injury victims—is provided through public and private health insurance plans. Moreover, the provision of medical care for all people is a major goal of public health, and the general public health effort to ensure access to health care for all through support of health care reform will be discussed later in the chapter. The public health effort to ensure health care for all must be viewed as a component of motor vehicle injury interventions that is supported by public health.

Child Passenger Safety

The principal interventions that have been supported by the research of the *Child Passenger Safety* initiative have concerned educating people about the need to use booster seats or seatbelts; providing car seats themselves to people with children, and advocating for safety seat laws and their enforcement. "There is strong evidence that child safety seat laws, safety seat distribution and education programs, communitywide education and enforcement campaigns, and incentive-plus-education programs are effective in increasing child safety seat use" (CDC, 2010b, para. 4).

Educating parents to use car seats and seat belts for their children is a pervasive theme in the interventions used to prevent child passenger injuries. The program, Protect the Ones You Love, is an example. The *Child Passenger Safety* Web site contains materials that can be used in educational campaigns including information about the risk of injury and tips for parents about how to keep their child safe in a motor vehicle:

> We all want to keep our children safe and secure and help them live to their full potential. Knowing how to prevent leading causes of child injury, like road traffic injuries, is a step toward this goal. Every hour, 150 children between ages 0 and 19 are treated in emergency departments for injuries sustained in motor vehicle crashes. More children ages 5–19 die from crash-related injuries than from any other type of injury. Thankfully, parents can play a key role in protecting the children they love from road traffic injuries.
>
> Prevention tips: One of the best protective measures you can take is using seat belts, child safety seats, and booster seats that are appropriate for your child's age and weight.

> *Know the Stages*
> - Typically, babies should be placed in rear facing car seats until they are at least 1 year old and weigh 20 pounds.
> - When babies move into front-facing car seats, they should remain in these seats until they are at least 4 years old or weigh 40 pounds.
> - Children should be seated in booster seats from about age 4 to age 8, or until they reach 4'9" tall.
> - All children ages 12 and under should be seated in the back seat of vehicles.
> - Helmets can help children. They should wear motorcycle or bike helmets any time they are on a motorcycle or bicycle." (CDC, 2010f, para. 1–6).

However, education alone has not been found effective. The Task Force on Community Preventive Services (TFCPS, 2005) did not find evidence that education programs that provide information to parents, children, or professional groups about the importance of child safety seats and how to use them properly were effective when used alone. A caveat is that the Task Force also said that evidence was insufficient because the educational interventions evaluated in their studies varied widely and the small number of available studies produced inconsistent results. The Task Force did find, however, that incentive and education programs that reward parents for obtaining and correctly using child safety seats or directly reward children for correctly using safety seats are effective, and these programs also include educational components.

There is also a substantial public health effort to change the social and physical environments to prevent child passenger injuries and fatalities. These efforts include "child safety seat laws, safety seat distribution and eduation programs, community-wide education and enforcement campaigns, and incentive-plus-education programs are effective in increasing child safety seat use" (CDC, 2010b, para. 4).

The TFCPS (2005) identified and rated the evidence on effectiveness for several interventions of this type. Child safety seat laws require children traveling in motor vehicles to be buckled into federally approved infant or child safety seats that are appropriate for the child's age and size. All states currently have child safety seat laws in place. The laws, which vary from state to state, specify the children they cover in terms of age, height, weight, or a combination of these factors. The Task Force found:

- "Child safety seat laws are effective in reducing fatal injuries to children by approximately 35%.
- These laws are also effective in reducing all injuries to children by approximately 17%.
- These laws are also effective in increasing child safety seat use by approximately 13 percentage points" (2005, p. 334).

Other interventions that public health advocates to change the social or physical environments to prevent childhood motor vehicle injuries and fatalities are

- "Distribution and education programs provide free or low-cost child safety seats to parents, along with education about proper use of the seats. The idea behind such programs is that parents who cannot afford a safety seat or who have a poor understanding of the importance of the seat might be more likely to use it if they receive financial help in acquiring a safety seat and learn about the importance of using it" (TFCPS, 2005, p. 335).
- Communitywide information and enhanced enforcement campaigns provide information about child safety seats and child automobile safety to an entire community (usually defined geographically). These campaigns use

several approaches: mass media, publicity, safety seat displays in public places, and special law enforcement strategies, such as checkpoints, dedicated law enforcement officials, or alternative penalties (e.g., warnings instead of tickets)" (2005, p. 337).

Teen Drivers

Similar to the *Child Passenger Safety* initiative, *Teen Drivers* also emphasizes education, and in addition, advocates for changes in the environment that will reduce the risk of injury and death among teen drivers.

Common types of educationally oriented interventions to promote safe teen driving include school-based instructional programs, peer organizations, and social norming campaigns (Elder et al., 2005). They generally focus on prevention of driving after drinking (DD) and riding with drinking drivers (RDD). A review of the effectiveness of various kinds of programs summarizes each type of program:

School-based instructional programs are a commonly used approach to addressing the problems of DD and RDD. These programs vary widely in their focus, with some targeting a variety of consequences of substance use and others more directly focused on problems related to alcohol-impaired driving. . . . Many of the more recent school-based programs to prevent DD and RDD are either explicitly theory based or incorporate theory-based concepts and methods, such as peer intervention social deviance, educational inoculation, and risk skills training. . . .

Social norming programs generally consist of ongoing, multiyear public information programs conducted on college campuses to reduce alcohol use, although they can also be conducted in other settings and for other target behaviors. The premise underlying the social norming approach is that students overestimate the amount and frequency of alcohol use among other students, and that this misperception influences them to drink more than they would otherwise. The key objective is to provide students with more objective normative information regarding student alcohol consumption, thus reducing their misperceptions and ultimately changing their behavior. Often this information is gathered via campus surveys, and then conveyed to students via campus media programs. In addition to such media programs, some social norming programs implement more instructional activities involving peer-to-peer interaction. . . .

School-based peer organizations are groups of students, often with faculty advisors, who encourage other students to refrain from drinking, DD, and RDD. The most widespread peer organization in the United States is Students Against Destructive Decisions (SADD), formerly called Students Against Drunk Driving. SADD activities, including assembly presentations, a curriculum with as many as 15 sessions, various school and community events, and a "Contract for Life" in which a student agrees to call a parent if he or she has been drinking or if the person responsible for driving has been drinking. SADD programs and curricula include activities aimed at providing information, influencing attitudes, and changing social norms. They include both didactic and interactive delivery, usually involving peer-to-peer delivery, but frequently involving outside experts as well" (Elder et al., 2005, pp. 290–294).

Three examples of programs demonstrate the variety of methods used in these types of interventions, but their common focus on changing individual teens' behavior related to safe driving through educational initiatives:

- A campuswide public awareness program was developed to provide objective information regarding student use of alcohol. The phrase "74% of University of Albany students drink once a week or less" provided the primary message.
- A 1 hour peer theater session, using trained peer "actors" and involving the audience in discussions regarding topical scenarios that were acted out.
- A program using Bandura's social learning theory and concept of self efficacy, which taught knowledge, attitudes, and judgments related to safe driving. A "reasoned argument" approach that minimized fear appeals was used. There was a focus on building self-efficacy with interactive sessions and role playing (Elder et al., 2005).

Educational programs may also focus on parents' role in teen driving. For instance, the Checkpoints Program is designed to improve parental management of the process of learning to drive, in driver's education classes. "It is the only intervention of its type with proven efficacy in increasing parental restrictions on newly licensed teen drivers. The effectiveness of this intervention will be evaluated by measuring the level of restrictions that parents place on their teens as they move from learner's permit to provisional license to full licensure. The number of violations and crashes among participating teens may also be measured" (CDC, 2010g, para. 1).

Interventions that target the larger social and physical environments include advocacy for building safer motor vehicles, enforcement of laws related to DD, and changing community attitudes about teen driving.

Regarding laws and law enforcement, lowering blood alcohol concentrations laws for young or inexperienced drivers; instituting sobriety checkpoints; and raising the minimum legal drinking age (MLDA) laws to 21 years of age (or maintain the age at 21 years) have all been found effective in reducing fatalities and injuries among teen drivers and their passengers. For example, "raising the MLDA is effective in reducing fatal injury crashes by approximately 17% and fatal and nonfatal injury crashes combined by approximately 15%. Lowering the MLDA leads to approximately an 8% increase in fatal injury crashes and approximately a 5% increase in fatal and nonfatal injury crashes combined" (TFCPS, 2005, p. 350). These legal interventions are strongly advocated by public health.

A current important public health advocacy issue related to teen driving is graduated driver licensing (GDL), a system of laws and practices that gradually introduce young drivers into the driving population. Full licensing is delayed while the teen gets initial driving experiences under low-risk conditions. GDL is associated with reductions of 38% and 40% in fatal and injury crashes, respectively, among 16-year-old drivers. A recent symposium, whose proceedings were published in *Injury Prevention* (Simons-Morton & Hartos, 2002), provided evidence about GDL:

Traditional driver education is insufficient for reducing the high risk of teen crashes (Mayhew & Simpson, pp. ii3–ii8).

■ Most traditional driver education provides classroom training about the rules of the road and a few hours of behind-the-wheel training. Research suggests that this approach is not effective in reducing the crash risk among newly licensed teen drivers. Driver education programs may be improved by teaching psychomotor, perceptual, and cognitive skills that are critical for safe driving, and by addressing inexperience, risky behaviors, and other age-related factors that increase the crash risk among young drivers. However, more research into these factors is needed before they can be addressed effectively.

Important risk factors highlight the need for graduated driver licensing (Williams & Ferguson, pp. ii9–ii16).

■ Young, beginning drivers have an extremely high-crash risk. Certain situations contribute to even greater risk, most notably nighttime driving and driving with teen passengers. The GDL approach addresses the high risks faced by young drivers by requiring an apprenticeship of planned and supervised practice, followed by a provisional license that places temporary restrictions on unsupervised driving in some higher risk situations.

Developmental characteristics of young drivers may contribute to their crash risk (Arnett, pp. ii17–ii23).

■ Inexperience increases the crash risk for new drivers of all ages. However, younger novice drivers crash at higher rates than older novice drivers. These higher crash rates may be due in part to developmental factors such as peer influence, poor perception of risk, and high emotionality. Research about such developmental characteristics could increase our understanding about why young drivers have higher crash rates and could help to improve driver education programs and licensing policies.

Greater parental involvement is needed (Simons-Morton et al., pp. ii24–31).

■ A growing body of research indicates that close parental management of teen drivers can lead to less risky driving behavior, fewer traffic tickets, and fewer crashes. However, many parents tend to be less involved than they could be. A recent study indicates that parents can be motivated to increase restrictions on their newly licensed teens, at least during the critical first few months of licensure. A model intervention, the Checkpoint Program, led to increased parental limits on teenage driving at licensure and 3 months after licensure.

GDL works (McKnight & Peck, pp. ii32–ii38).

■ GDL has consistently proven effective in reducing new driver crash risk. Although research is still needed to better understand which components of GDL are essential, it remains a promising solution for improving teen driver safety. It may also provide the best context for improving driver education and increasing parental involvement, both of which could also reduce the crash risk for teen drivers" (Simon-Morton & Hartos, 2002).

Media campaigns are usually the method of attempting to influence community norms, values, and beliefs about teen driving. These include the seasonal educational campaigns sponsored by the CDC to raise awareness and change community attitudes: National Child Passenger Safety Week, National Teen Driver Safety Week, National Drunk and Drugged Driving Prevention Month, and Native American Road Safety

(CDC, 2010f). Another example is the CDC sponsored national Teen Safe Driving Campaign, which Ogilvy Public Relations Worldwide will develop to improve the safety of teen drivers, their passengers, and other drivers. The campaign will emphasize the benefits of "practice driving with a parent in the car; increase parents' awareness of the highest risks for teen drivers; redirect parental monitoring to high-risk behaviors; increase the number of parents who monitor their teen's driving; and increase parents' awareness of graduated driver licensing (GDL) laws in their state" (CDC, 2010g, para. 14).

The TFCPS (2005) found strong evidence of effectiveness of mass media campaigns. They have been found to be effective in decreasing all crashes by approximately 13% and injury crashes by approximately 10%:

> Mass media campaigns are typically carried out in conjunction with other programs and policies to prevent alcohol-impaired driving. Where adequate local resources can support a mass media campaign that is carefully planned, well executed, attains adequate audience exposure, and is supported by other prevention activities, this combination of activities can be effective in reducing alcohol-impaired driving" (TFCPS, 2005, p. 360).

Some interventions combine teen education and communitywide media campaigns, such as the community-based intervention to increase seat belt use among teens in Mississippi, where "Meharry Medical College and Jackson State University are evaluating the independent and combined effects of a multifaceted, communitywide campaign to increase seatbelt usage among adolescent motorists ages 15–19 in Jackson, Mississippi. The project aims to: (a) evaluate the impact of a targeted, school-based, peer-to-peer, service learning intervention; (b) evaluate the impact of a comprehensive, community-based, educational and media campaign to increase youth awareness and usage of seat belts; and (c) compare study results with other secondary data sets that reflect changes in teen seat belt use rates" (CDC, 2010g , para. 5).

CHILDHOOD OBESITY

Obesity is a worldwide problem, which is more and more frequently beginning in childhood. In the United States, the Division of Nutrition, Physical Activity, and Obesity (DNPAO) is the CDC's lead division for obesity prevention and control. The DNPAO is at the forefront in the development of knowledge about obesity—its prevalence, incidence, risk factors, causes, and consequences. This information, then, is being used to develop prevention interventions—primary, secondary, and tertiary. The following description of public health practice related to the prevention and control of obesity is taken mainly from the CDC (CDC, 2010c), which again is the predominant actor in terms of agenda setting, surveillance and research, and source of funding to stimulate prevention strategies. The emphasis is on childhood obesity.

Surveillance and Research

Overweight and obesity are defined by the WHO as "abnormal or excessive fat accumulation that may impair health" (WHO, 2010). There are a number of methods of measuring obesity and overweight. These include skinfold thickness measurements (with calipers), underwater weighing, bioelectrical impedance, dual-energy x-ray absorptiometry (DXA), and isotope dilution. However, these methods are expensive and, in addition, need to be performed with expensive equipment by highly trained personnel. Further, many of them can be difficult to standardize across observers or machines, making comparisons across studies and time periods difficult and unreliable (CDC, 2010j).

As a result, the body mass index (BMI) is commonly used in studies of overweight and obesity in populations and individuals although it is not as accurate as more expensive measures of obesity and overweight. BMI is a simple index of weight-to-height that is calculated as the weight of an individual in kilograms divided by the square of the height in meters (kg/m2).

"BMI provides the most useful population-level measure of overweight and obesity as it is the same for both sexes and for all ages of adults. However, it should be considered as a rough guide because it may not correspond to the same degree of fatness in different individuals.

The new WHO Child Growth Standards, launched in April 2006, include BMI charts for infants and young children up to age 5. However, measuring overweight and obesity in children aged 5 to 14 years is challenging because there is not a standard definition of childhood obesity applied worldwide. WHO is currently developing an international growth reference for school-age children and adolescents" (WHO, 2010, para. 3 & 5).

The BMI is calculated for children and adults in the same way, but the criteria used to interpret the BMI for children and adolescents are different from those for adults. For children, overweight and obesity use age- and sex-specific growth charts. These growth charts are a series of percentile curves that illustrate the distribution of selected body measurements in children and have been used to track the growth of infants, children, and adolescents in the United States since 1977. See Figure 5.1 for an example of a growth chart. The reasons for using age- and sex-specific percentiles from growth charts to determine overweight and obesity in children are that the amount of body fat changes with age; and the amount of body fat differs between girls and boys.

In the United States, the CDC recommends the use of the WHO growth standards to monitor growth for infants and children ages 0 to 2 years of age and the CDC growth charts for children age 2 years and older. Using these growth charts:

■ Overweight is defined as a BMI at or above the 85th percentile and lower than the 95th percentile.
■ Obesity is defined as a BMI at or above the 95th percentile for children of the same age and sex (CDC, 2010j).

As with other public health efforts, data systems are necessary to provide information about the incidence, prevalence, and risk factors for obesity; to conduct research on the causes and consequences of obesity; and to evaluate the effectiveness of interventions aimed at preventing and controlling obesity. Surveillance data for obesity is obtained from the NCHS, (2010a).

The National Health and Nutrition Examination Survey (NHANES) is a program of studies designed to assess the health and nutritional status of adults and children in the United States. The survey is unique in that it combines interviews and physical examinations. NHANES is a major program of the National Center for Health Statistics (NCHS). NCHS is part of the Centers for Disease Control and Prevention (CDC) and has the responsibility for producing vital and health statistics for the Nation.

The NHANES program began in the early 1960s and has been conducted as a series of surveys focusing on different population groups or health topics. In 1999, the survey became a continuous program that has a changing focus on various health and nutrition measurements to meet

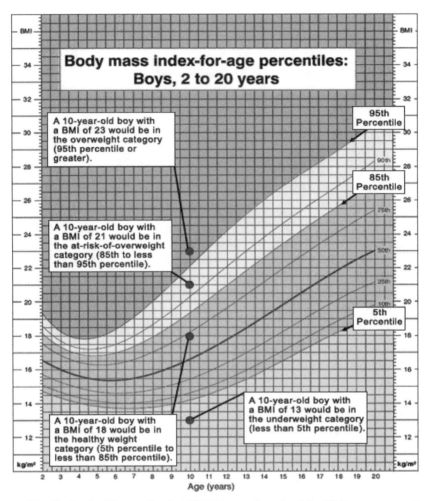

Body mass index-for-age percentiles:
Boys, 2 to 20 years

A 10-year-old boy with a BMI of 23 would be in the overweight category (95th percentile or greater).

95th Percentile

85th Percentile

A 10-year-old boy with a BMI of 21 would be in the at-risk-of-overweight category (85th to less than 95th percentile).

5th Percentile

A 10-year-old boy with a BMI of 13 would be in the underweight category (less than 5th percentile).

A 10-year-old boy with a BMI of 18 would be in the healthy weight category (5th percentile to less than 85th percentile).

Age (years)

- The Center for Disease Control (CDC) has categorized the BMI measurement within the United States so that a clear and distinct definition of obesity can be ascertained

- This categorization of the BMI measurement's criteria can be adjusted according to age, gender, or race

FIGURE 5.1   Body Mass Index

emerging needs. The survey examines a nationally representative sample of about 5,000 persons each year. These persons are located in counties across the country, 15 of which are visited each year.

The NHANES interview includes demographic, socioeconomic, dietary, and health-related questions. The examination component consists of medical, dental, and physiological measurements, as well as laboratory tests administered by highly trained medical personnel.

Findings from this survey will be used to determine the prevalence of major diseases and risk factors for diseases. Information will be used to assess nutritional status and its association with health promotion and disease prevention. NHANES findings are also the basis for national standards for such measurements as height, weight, and blood pressure. Data from this survey will be used in epidemiological studies and health sciences research, which help develop sound public health policy, direct and design health programs and services, and expand the health knowledge for the Nation. (NCHS, 2010a, para. 1–4)

DNPAO also has two surveillance systems that are program-based: Pediatric Nutrition Surveillance System (PedNSS) and Pregnancy Surveillance System (PNSS). Both are used to monitor the nutritional status of low income infants, children, and women in federally funded maternal and child health programs. PedNSS provides data on the prevalence and trends of nutrition-related problems. PNSS is used to identify risk factors associated with infant mortality and poor birth outcomes. The data sources for PedNSS and PNSS are existing data from the following public health programs for nutrition surveillance:

- Special Supplemental Nutrition Program for Women, Infants, and Children (WIC)
- Early and Periodic Screening, Diagnosis, and Treatment (EPSDT) Program (PedNSS only)
- Title V Maternal and Child Health Program (MCH)

Besides surveillance related to nutrition, physical activity, and obesity, DNPAO supports special studies to evaluate and enhance the effectiveness of physical activity and nutrition programs. For example, current research topics include the following:

- Effectiveness of parent-focused strategies to reduce the time children spend watching television
- Influences of the home environment on sugar-sweetened beverage consumption
- Use of policy interventions to promote physical activity
- Effectiveness of breastfeeding interventions in various settings

Based on the surveillance and research conducted or sponsored by DNPAO and other groups, we know a great deal about the extent of the childhood obesity problem, as we shall discuss now.

The CDC has reported that a third of the children in America are obese. Childhood obesity is becoming an epidemic in developed nations as well as in the United States. Childhood obesity has affected every demographic population within the United States and this problem is becoming a global concern. The problem is considered pandemic as a result of the global distribution of childhood obesity, but because incident rates continue to increase, it is not thought to be endemic (Kimm & Obarzanek, 2002).

Studies have shown that the average BMI of the American youth has increased 12% since 1963. In chart format, the average BMI in 1963 was 21.3 and the current BMI is 24.1 (LaFontaine, 2008). The NHANES, has calculated that the incidence of childhood obesity has tripled since 1980 (LaFontaine).

According to the CDC's charts, the incidence of childhood obesity in children 2–5 years of age has increased from 5.0% in 1980 to 13.9% in 2004 (Ogden et al., 2006). Children in the 6–11 age bracket and the 12–19 age bracket have seen increases of childhood obesity since 1980. The 6–11 age group saw an increase in childhood obesity from 5.0% in 1980 to 13.9% in 2004. The 12–19 age group had an increase from 6.6% in 1980 to 18.8% in 2004. Adolescents 12–19 years of age saw the largest increase with an obesity incidence of 5% in 1980 to 17.4% in 2004 (Ogden et al., 2006).

The prevalence of childhood obesity (see Figure 5.2) has also been increasing over the past 4 decades. Data tabulated by the CDC determine how many children are overweight and obese.

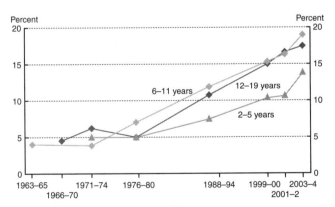

Note: Overweight is defined as BM >= gender- and weight-specific 95th percentile from the 2000 CDC Growth Charts.
Source: National Health Examination Surveys II (ages 6–11) and III (ages 12–17). National Health and Nutrition Examination Survevs I. II. III and 1999–2004. NCHS. CDC.

FIGURE 5.2   Trends in Childhood Obesity

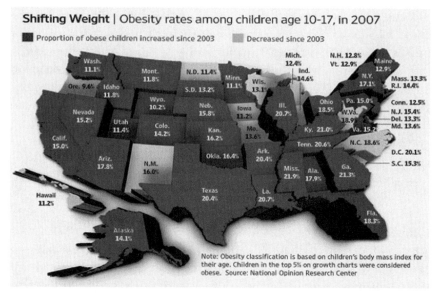

Note: Obesity classification is based on children's body mass index for their age. Children in the top 5% on growth charts were considered obese. Source: National Opinion Research Center

- Nationwide, roughly 17% of school-age children are obese and an estimated 33% are overweight according to the Centers for Disease Control

- This state-by-state map is based on children's body mass index (BMI) for their age. Children in their top 5% on growth charts were considered obese

- According to this map, at 21.9%, Mississippi had the highest obesity rate in the U.S. in 2007

FIGURE 5.3   Childhood Obesity in the U.S.

The CDC determined that the prevalence of children being overweight had gone from 13% in the 1970s to 33% in 2004 (Ogden et al., 2006). These data indicate that in 2004 one third of all children in United States were overweight or obese (see Figure 5.3; CDC, 2009).

In addition to studies of prevalence and incidence, the CDC has been investigating possible causes of the increase in childhood obesity. Multiple studies have shown a strong correlation between childhood obesity and parental obesity. There appears to be a familial link in that children of parents who were obese as kids tend to have high BMIs (Li, Law, Lo Conte, & Power, 2009). Studies have also indicated that obese children maintain and increase their BMI scores in adulthood to become obese adults (Serdula et al., 1993). One study monitored approximately 16 million students 13–20 years of age and found that only 14.7% reduced their weight below the 95th percentile, which represents the obesity level

(Gordon-Larsen, 2004). Another study found that approximately 80% of overweight children 10–15 years of age become obese by 25 (Whitaker, Wright, Pepe, Seidel, & Dietz, 1997).

Childhood obesity is occurring throughout the world.

The International Obesity Task Force (IOTF) has utilized the BMI to determine the number of children who are obese globally (see Figure 5.4).

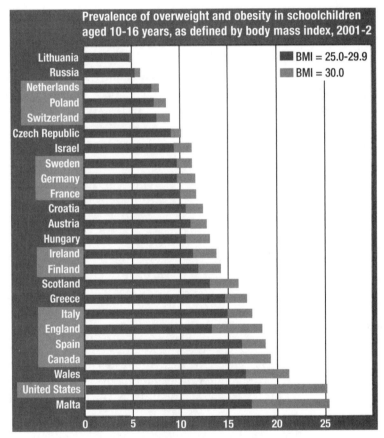

- The International Obesity Task Force estimates that there are 30–45 million children aged 5–17 who are obese around the world (International Obesity Taskforce)

- The task force expanded the research to include children that are under 5 and found that 22 million of these children were overweight (World Health Organization)

FIGURE 5.4   Global Distribution of Childhood Obesity

The organization estimates that 30–45 million children 5–17 years of age are obese (IOTF, 2009). The task force expanded the research to include children who were under 5 years old and found that 22 million of these children were overweight (World Health Organization [WHO], 2009 International Association for the Study of Obesity, 2010). The interpretation of these data suggests that childhood obesity is a global problem, thus supporting the assertion that childhood obesity is pandemic.

Childhood obesity is usually associated with living in developed nations. The United States is ranked as the 9th most obese nation in the world (WHO, 2010a). Nations that have similar socioeconomic characteristics rank as high as the United States in prevalence of childhood obesity. Overall, childhood obesity appears to be a problem of developed countries such as England, Australia, and the United States. In addition, childhood obesity rates seem to be climbing in these nations. For example, BMI measurements in England between 2000 and 2004 increased for English boys from 20% to 25% ("Global Trends," 2008).

However, there has been an increase in childhood obesity in developing nations such as Thailand (Dehghan, Akhtarr-Danesh, & Merchant, 2005). Thailand experienced an increase in childhood obesity from 12.2% to 16.6% in only 2 years (2009). Developing countries tend to have difficulty in reporting credible BMI data to the WHO because few studies of childhood obesity are conducted, and those that are conducted often have data collection problems. Nevertheless, credible findings are suggested.

Poor nations rarely have a problem with childhood obesity, overall. However, developing nations tend to report higher obesity rates among children of the wealthy. The childhood obesity studies have also shown that wealthy societies typically have higher rates of childhood obesity. This seemingly paradoxical finding is explained by the socioeconomic status of the children (Khan & Bowman, 1999). Lower socioeconomic status children in wealthy nations are at greater risk for obesity than children of higher socioeconomic status in these nations. Conversely, children of high socioeconomic status in poor nations are at the greatest risk for obesity in these nations.

In the United States, lower socioeconomic status is one of the most important risk factors associated with childhood obesity, as is minority race and/or ethnicity (see Figure 5.5). African-Americans, Hispanics, and Native Americans have the highest rates of childhood obesity in the United

Risk Factors

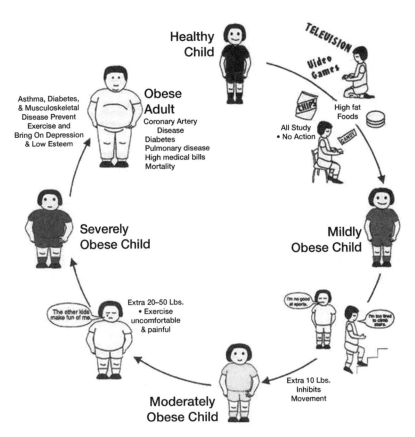

- Diet is one of the major risk factors of childhood obesity

- A poor diet will lead to an increase in BMI as a result of excess fat

- The socioeconomic status of a child is one of the most important risk factors associated with childhood obesity

- Nurture is another risk factor for childhood obesity

FIGURE 5.5   The Vicious Cycle of Childhood Obesity

States. The explanation for the associations between socioeconomic status, race and ethnicity, and childhood obesity is generally understood to be highly related to nutrition: fewer healthy choices in supermarkets in low income, minority neighborhoods, more eating at fast food restaurants because of convenience and availability, and the high cost of more nutritious, lower calorie foods.

Lack of physical activity is another important risk factor for childhood obesity (see Figure 5.6). Coupled with poor eating habits, a sedentary life style is highly likely to lead to excessive weight gain. Research indicates that children spend nearly 3 years of their waking hours watching television (Robinson, 1998; Hu, Li, Colditz, Willet, & Manson, 2003). This behavior has led to a sedentary lifestyle. The adverse effect of television-watching on physical activity is compounded by the accompanying exposure to advertising for poor food choices such as sweetened beverages and breakfast foods. Other technologies such as video games further reduce the time children in the United States spend in physical activity.

Parental behavior is another risk factor for childhood obesity. Children tend to learn their eating habits from their parents. A child's risk of becoming obese doubles if one or both of the parents are obese (IOM, 2004). On the other hand, parents can influence children to eat healthily by setting an example and providing nutritious meals at home. In addition, schools can have a large impact on food choices, which impact childhood obesity for better or worse. A school cafeteria that provides a soda vending machine is enabling a child to make a poor choice.

Like many physical conditions, obesity may have a genetic component. One theory links an imbalance in the hormone Leptin to excess weight (Strauss, 2000). Leptin is believed to regulate the storage of body fat, and an imbalance of this hormone would increase the ability of the body to store adipose tissue. The imbalance is believed to be of genetic origin, and thus, the risk factor would be familial.

The increased number of obese children in the United States has resulted in an increased prevalence of serious medical conditions in this population. Diseases that were once considered adult problems are now being diagnosed in obese children including diseases of the kidneys, pancreas, heart, and circulatory system. Pediatricians have become accustomed to treating diseases in the child population that were previous prevalent only in adults, and the childhood obesity epidemic has changed the practice of pediatrics, such that pediatricians now commonly treat type II diabetes, hypertension, elevated cholesterol, and hyperlipidemia. Obese children have been found to have an increased risk of type II diabetes (Trevino, Fogt, Wyatt, Vasquez, & Sosa, 2008). The circulatory system of the obese child is also affected. Obese children are more likely than non-obese children to have elevated cholesterol, hypertension, and hyperlipidemia (Freedman, Khan, Dietz, Srinivasan, & Berenson, 2001). Although childhood imparts

Risk Factors

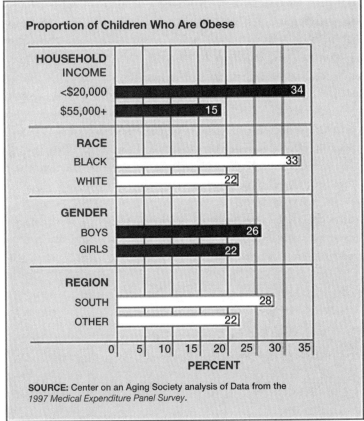

Proportion of Children Who Are Obese

FIGURE 5.6   Risk Factors for Childhood Obesity

- The actual place where a child is raised could be a risk factor for childhood obesity

- In the U.S, Native Americans, African Americans, and Hispanics have a higher prevalence of obesity

- Asians and Pacific Islanders have lower rates of obesity

- Lack of physical activity and a sedentary lifestyle will result in excessive weight gain when coupled with a poor eating regimen

certain immunity to the young heart, the consistent elevation of the LDL cholesterol throughout childhood is likely to result in cardiovascular problems later in life. Hypertension, or high blood pressure, stresses the heart because the heart muscle has to work harder to pump blood throughout the body. Obesity in childhood increases the amount of time throughout the lifespan in which the heart is undergoing stress. Children who are obese also suffer from hyperlipidemia, an excess of fat in the blood, at a higher rate than non-obese children. The circulatory system exerts more effort to move blood through the body as a result of hyperlipidemia. These three disorders have a major effect on the heart later in the obese child's life. The circulatory system may be adversely affected as a result of these conditions, which will cause the heart to work longer and harder. A child with these conditions will have an increased likelihood of adult heart and circulatory problems.

In addition to physical health problems, childhood obesity has a negative impact on social relationships and sense of well-being. Not surprisingly, research has found that obese children are at greater risk than their non-obese counterparts of having low social status in school (McNeely, 2008; Friedlander, Larkin, Rosen, Palermo, & Redline, 2003). They are more likely to be the targets of bullying, teasing, and scorn, which have long-term emotional consequences including depression and low self-esteem (Moran, 1999).

Interventions

A major partnership for developing interventions to prevent and control childhood obesity is the Nutrition, Physical Activity and Obesity Program (NPAO), a cooperative agreement between the DNPAO and 23 state health departments. NPAO's goal is to prevent and control obesity and other chronic diseases through healthful eating and physical activity. "The state programs develop strategies to leverage resources and coordinate statewide efforts with multiple partners to address all of the following DNPAO principal target areas:

■ Increase physical activity
■ Increase the consumption of fruits and vegetables
■ Decrease the consumption of sugar sweetened beverages
■ Increase breastfeeding initiation, duration and exclusivity
■ Reduce the consumption of high energy dense foods
■ Decrease television viewing" (CDC, 2010c)

The most authoritative public health plan for preventing and controlling obesity has been developed by the CDC. Notably, the strategies are aimed at changing the social and physical environments at the local level. It is very much a community-based plan to ensure that there are opportunities and incentives for all to obtain nutritious food and engage in physical activity, thereby addressing the underlying causes of obesity. The strategies do not rely on education alone. Rather they are implemented through policy changes and partnerships with local organizations. As the authors write, "This product is the result of an innovative and collaborative process that seeks to reverse the U.S. obesity epidemic by transforming communities into places where healthy lifestyle choices are easily incorporated into everyday life. To reverse the obesity epidemic, we must change our physical and food environments to provide more opportunities for people to eat healthy foods and to be physically active on a daily basis" (Keener, Goodman, Lowry, Zaro, & Kettel Khan, 2009).

The 24 strategies, which the CDC recommends to encourage and support healthy lives, are contained in Table 5.2. Each strategy is illustrated by a community-based example of its implementation.

IMPROVING ACCESS TO MEDICAL CARE

Access to quality health care is essential to secondary and tertiary prevention, and therefore, to public health. Without timely and adequate health care, an acute health problem, such as an injury, that if treated appropriately would have no long-term consequences, becomes a chronic condition and a chronic condition, such as diabetes, is exacerbated. When primary prevention fails and people sustain injuries or become obese—the subjects of the previous sections—they require access to health care. However, the United States is the only wealthy nation that does not guarantee at least a basic level of health care for its citizens. As a result, public health advocates universal health coverage, or as it is often called, health care reform.

The history of health care reform in the United States is long and tortuous. Debate over reform has recurred with regularity since the early part of the 20th century. There have been many failed attempts to achieve universal coverage. In 1912, Teddy Roosevelt and his Progressive Party endorsed social insurance, including health insurance. In 1915, the American Association for Labor Legislation published a draft bill for compulsory health insurance, which was not enacted. In 1939, Senator Wagner introduced the National Health Bill in Congress, which did not get out of committee. In 1944, President Franklin Roosevelt identified medical care as a right in his State of the Union address. The Social Security Board called for compulsory national health coverage a few months later in 1945. President Truman took

TABLE 5.2   Strategies to Prevent and Control Obesity Through Community-Based Changes in the Environment

Category 1: Strategies to promote the availability of affordable healthy food and beverages
Strategy 1: Increase availability of healthier food and beverage choices in public service venues
Community Example
■ In St. Paul, Minnesota, the "Five a Day Power Plus Program" increased the variety of fruits and vegetables offered in schools by providing an additional fruit item on days baked desserts were served, promoting fruits and vegetables at point-of-purchase, and enhancing the attractiveness of fruits and vegetables. Evaluation of the program found that fruit and vegetable consumption increased significantly among children in the intervention group as compared with a control group (Perry et al., 1998).
Strategy 2: Improve availability of affordable healthier food and beverage choices in public service venues
Community Example
■ The New York City Department of Health operates the Health Bucks Program to make fruits and vegetables more affordable to residents who receive food stamps. For every five dollars' worth of food stamps spent at farmers' markets, individuals receive a $2 Health Bucks coupon which can be redeemed year round at more than 30 farmers' markets citywide. In 2007, the City Health Department reported that New Yorkers used more than 40% of the 9,000 Health Bucks distributed in 2006 (New York City Department of Health and Mental Hygiene, 2007).
Strategy 3: Improve geographic availability of supermarkets in underserved areas
Community Example
■ The Philadelphia Food Marketing Task Force investigated the lack of supermarkets in Philadelphia and released 10 recommendations to increase the number of supermarkets in Philadelphia's underserved communities. A new funding initiative was created using public funds to leverage supermarket development. To date, the initiative has committed $67 million in funding for 69 supermarket projects in 27 Pennsylvania counties, creating or preserving 3,900 jobs (Burton & Duane, 2004).
Strategy 4: Provide incentives to food retailers to locate in and/or offer healthier food and beverage choices in underserved areas
Community Example
■ The city of Richmond, California, attracted a national discount grocery store to an urban retail center with adjacent affordable housing by offering an attractive incentive package, which included land sold at a reduced cost to the developer; a Federal Urban Development Action Grant of $3.5 million for commercial development; a zoning designation that provided tax incentives; assistance in negotiations with State regulatory agencies; improvements to surrounding sidewalks, streetscape, and traffic signals; and concessions on design standards (PolicyLink & Bay Area Local Initiatives Support Corporation, 2008).

Category 1: Strategies to promote the availability of affordable healthy food and beverages

Strategy 5: Improve availability of mechanisms for purchasing foods from farms

Community Example

■ In 2005, Jefferson Elementary School, in Riverside, California, launched a farm-to-school salad bar program which provides elementary school students access to a daily salad bar stocked with a variety of locally grown produce as an alternative to the standard hot lunch. Two small, locally owned family farms, within 30 miles of the school, sell their produce at an affordable price and make weekly deliveries to the school. Since implementing the farm-to-school salad bar program, the Riverside school district has expanded the program to four additional elementary schools (Anupama, Kalb, & Beery, 2006).

Strategy 6: Provide incentives for the production, distribution, and procurement of foods from local farms

Community Example

■ The Hartford Food System (HFS) in Connecticut is a nonprofit organization working to create an equitable and sustainable food system that addresses the underlying causes of hunger and poor nutrition facing low-income and elderly residents. In addition to developing innovative projects and initiatives that tackle food cost, access, and nutrition, the organization actively participates in public policy initiatives aimed at increasing production, distribution, and procurement of foods from local farms at the local, State, and Federal Government levels (Feenstra, 1997).

Category 2: Strategies to support healthy food and beverage choices

Strategy 7: Restrict availability of less healthy foods and beverages in public service venues

Community Example

■ The city of Baldwin Park, California, established nutrition standards for all snack foods and beverages sold in over 30 after school programs (including snack offerings in vending machines). The afterschool nutrition standards primarily focus on eliminating less healthy snacks and beverages that exceed recommended fat, calorie, and sugar intake for school-aged children (Healthy Eating Active Communities, 2007).

Strategy 8: Institute smaller portion size options in public service venues

Community Example

Although the following example describes a program that target private restaurants, it may serve as a model for local communities that wish to promote greater access to healthy portion sizes in public service venues.

■ The Texas Department of State Health Services developed the *Tex Plate* program to assist Texas restaurants in serving healthier portion sizes to consumers. Participating restaurants receive specialized 9-inch plates that indicate proper portions of key food groups such as vegetables, protein, and whole grains. The program is designed to encourage participating restaurants to increase the vegetable portion of the meal and decrease the entrée and starch portions of the meal (Texas Department of State Health Services, 2008).

continued

TABLE 5.2   Strategies to Prevent and Control Obesity Through Community-Based Changes in the Environment (continued)

Category 2: Strategies to support healthy food and beverage choices

Strategy 9: Limit advertisements of less healthy foods and beverages

Community Example

■ The Mercedes Independent School District in Mercedes, Texas, adopted a comprehensive Student Nutrition/Wellness Plan in 2005 which includes a marketing component. The policy states that schools will promote healthy food choices and will not allow advertising that promotes less nutritious food choices. The plan also defines and prohibits possession of foods of minimal nutritional value at school (Mercedes Independent School District, 2005).

Strategy 10: Discourage consumption of sugar-sweetened beverages

Community Example

■ In 2002, the Los Angeles Unified School District adopted the Motion to Promote Healthy Beverage Sales. The motion bans the sale of soft drinks on school campuses; prohibits schools from entering into new or extended sales contracts of unapproved beverages; allows only approved beverages to be sold in vending machines, cafeterias, and student stores; monitors compliance through an audit program; disseminates information on healthy beverage sale options; and develops a new revenue model to make up for anticipated net loss of Associated Student Body monies related to the ban on soft drinks (LAUSD, 2002).

Category 3: Strategy to encourage breastfeeding

Strategy 11: Increase support for breastfeeding

Community Example

■ In 1998, California passed the *Breastfeeding at Work* law, which requires all employers to ensure that employees are provided with adequate facilities for breastfeeding or expressing milk. In 2002, the State passed *Lactation Accommodation*, which expands prior workplace provisions to require adequate break time and space for breastfeeding or milk expression, with a violation penalty of $100 (Shealy, Li, Benton-Davis, & Grummer-Strawn, 2005).

Category 4: Strategies to encourage physical activity or limit sedentary activity among children and youth

Strategy 12: Require physical education in schools

Community Example

■ In 2006, West Virginia enacted Senate Bill 785, which calls for the Department of Education to establish a requirement that every student enrolled in a public school participate in PE classes during the school year. The bill also specified participation times for PE classes by grade level. For example, elementary school students are required to participate in at least 30 minutes of PE class 3 days a week, middle school students are required to participate in at least one full period of PE each school day for a semester, and high school students are required to complete no less than one full course credit of PE class prior to graduation (Winterfeld, 2007).

Category 4: Strategies to encourage physical activity or limit sedentary activity among children and youth

Strategy 13: Increase the amount of physical activity in physical education programs in schools

Community Example

- Owensboro, Kentucky, overhauled its school-based PE curriculum after a study found that 60% of the Owensboro-area population was obese or overweight. A partnership was formed between the city's hospitals and schools and $750,000 was donated to equip 11 school-based fitness centers with treadmills, stationary bikes, rowing machines, and weightlifting stations. PE teachers were trained using "new PE" techniques, which stress the importance of keeping students physically active for at least 30-to 60-minute increments during class time (Weir, 2004).

- Equestrian Trails Elementary School, located in Wellington, Florida, received a STARS award from the National Association for Sport and Physical Education in recognition of its outstanding PE program. The PE staff at Equestrian Trails Elementary designed a yearly plan of instruction using physical activity and fitness components as the primary foundation for its curriculum. The curriculum teaches students the basic skills of several movement forms, including team, dual, and individual sports, and dance (National Association for Sport and Physical Education, n.d.).

Strategy 14: Increase opportunities for extracurricular physical activity

Community Example

- The city of Eugene, Oregon, and the Bethel School District pooled their resources to purchase and develop a 70-acre parcel of land. The property now includes a 35-acre site for Meadow View School and 35 acres for Bethel Community Park, which includes wetlands, a running path, ball fields, and a skate/community park. Many students can walk through the park to get to school (Oregon Transportation and Growth Management Program, 2005).

Strategy 15: Reduce screen time in public service venues

Community Example

- In 2006, the New York City Department of Health and Mental Hygiene Board of Health implemented an amendment to the New York City Health Code, which regulates group day care in New York City. The amended article prohibits television, video, and visual recordings for children younger than 2 years of age. In addition, television, video, and visual recordings are limited to 60 minutes per day of educational programming for children 2 years or older (New York City Department of Health and Mental Hygiene, 2006).

Category 5: Strategies to create safe communities that support physical activity

Strategy 16: Improve access to outdoor recreational facilities

Community Example

- KaBOOM! is a national nonprofit organization that empowers local communities to build playgrounds in neighborhoods that lack play spaces for children. The KaBOOM! process helps residents of local communities bring together the capacity, resources, volunteers, and planning needed to fulfill the vision of a great place to play within walking distance of every child in America. The KaBOOM! Web site provides information and resources for community residents to apply for a KaBOOM!-led playground build or to follow detailed steps to build their own playground.

continued

TABLE 5.2   Strategies to Prevent and Control Obesity Through Community-Based Changes in the Environment *(continued)*

Category 5: Strategies to create safe communities that support physical activity

Strategy 17: Enhance infrastructure supporting bicycling

Community Example

■ In May 2005, Boulder, Colorado, was awarded Gold status as a Bicycle-Friendly Community by the League of American Bicyclists. The city committed 15% of its annual transportation budget, $3.1 million, toward bicycle enhancement and maintenance activities. More than 95% of Boulder's arterial streets have bicycle facilities and all local and regional buses are equipped with bike racks. In addition, Boulder has created an online bike routing system that provides cyclists a direct and safe bike route to travel within city limits (League of American Bicyclists, 2005).

Strategy 18: Enhance infrastructure supporting walking

Community Example

■ In 2002, the City of Oakland, California, adopted a Pedestrian Master Plan which designates a network of pedestrian facilities and distinguishes segments and intersections in need of particular attention for safety enhancements. The city estimated pedestrian volumes throughout the city based on land use, population, and other network characteristics, and used these estimates in conjunction with crash data, traffic data, and community input to identify and prioritize areas with both safety problems and high pedestrian demand (City of Oakland, n.d.).

Strategy 19: Support locating schools within easy walking distance of residential areas

Community Example

■ In 2005, the City of Milwaukee began its Neighborhood Schools initiative. As a result of this initiative, the city decided to build six new schools from the ground up and spent millions of dollars revamping and expanding dilapidated schools that were located in and around community neighborhoods. The goals of the initiative were to reduce the number of students being bused to schools around the city and to increase the number of students walking or biking to schools that were centrally located and close to their neighborhoods (National Center for Safe Routes to School, 2007).

Strategy 20: Improve access to public transportation

Community Example

■ Local business owners and residents of the South Park neighborhood of Tucson, Arizona, received funding from the local government and the Federal Transit Administration (FTA) to implement a series of improvements to the existing public transit system. Funds were used to install six new artistic bus shelters, new traffic signals, and additional sidewalk and curb access ramps for public transit users, bicyclers, and pedestrians. As a result of the efforts to revitalize its public transit infrastructure, South Park has experienced renewed pride in its community and helped to rebuild its local economy (Public Transportation Partnership for Tomorrow, 2008).

Category 5: Strategies to create safe communities that support physical activity

Strategy 21: Zone for mixed-use development

Community Example

■ The concept of mixed-use development is the official growth management policy for Eugene, Oregon, which focuses on integrating mixed-use developments within the city's urban growth boundary. The city's regional transportation master plan targets dozens of potential "mixed-use centers" for development into quality neighborhoods that enjoy higher densities, more transportation options, and convenient access to shopping, consumer services, and basic amenities. By combining mixed-use centers with improved transit options, the plan aims to reduce dependence on automobile travel, encourage walking, and reduce the need for costly street improvements (City of Eugene, n.d.).

Strategy 22: Enhance personal safety in areas where persons are or could be physically active

Community Example

■ Detroit, Michigan, has one of the highest home foreclosure rates in the country, resulting in a dramatic increase in the number of abandoned buildings and boarded-up homes which attract vandals and petty crime. In response, Urban Farming, an international nonprofit organization, joined forces with the local county government to transform 20 abandoned properties into active fruit and vegetable garden plots that feed the homeless and improve the aesthetic appeal of city neighborhoods. Since establishing the gardens, residents report less vandalism and blight in their community and the local county government donates water to maintain the city gardens on an ongoing basis (Bear, 2008).

Strategy 23: Enhance traffic safety in areas where persons are or could be physically active

Community Example

■ In the mid-1990s, the City of West Palm Beach, Florida, adopted a downtown-wide traffic calming policy to improve street safety for nonmotorized users. The city's main streets were retrofitted with important pedestrian safety measures, including raised intersections, two-way streets, road narrowings and roundabouts to slow traffic, wide sidewalks, tree-lined streets, and shortened pedestrian crossings. As a result of these efforts, city streets are perceived as safe by pedestrians, property values more than doubled in the downtown area, and commercial retail space is 80% occupied (Lockwood & Stillings, 1998).

Category 6: Strategy to encourage communities to organize for change

Strategy 24: Participate in community coalitions or partnerships to address obesity

Community Example

■ PedNet Coalition in Columbia, Missouri, is a community coalition that includes 5,000 individuals and 75 businesses, government agencies, and nonprofit organizations. The goal of the coalition is to develop and restore a network of nature trails and urban "pedways" connecting residential subdivisions, worksites, shopping districts, parks, schools, and recreation centers (PedNet Coalition, 2008).

up the cause and was a strong advocate for national health reform after he took office in 1945. His election in 1948 seemed to be a mandate for health care reform. However, he failed, like those before him, in this case because of efforts to label the reform socialist.

Rather, health care benefits have been achieved piecemeal and inconsistently throughout the 20th century, covering some groups, but never all and providing us with the hodgepodge that we have today, whereby many people have no health insurance, and among those who have benefits, coverage ranges from inadequate to comprehensive—often within the same family. The greatest reforms came under President Lyndon Johnson in the 1960s, when Medicaid and Medicare were passed into law. Medicare, a federal program, provides basic health coverage for people over 65, regardless of their resources and health condition. Medicaid, a federal–state program, covers low income people who are uninsured. However, because each state has its own Medicaid program with unique eligibility criteria, people may qualify for Medicaid in one state, but not in another. Even after the passage of Medicare and Medicaid, many people were uninsured since for the remainder, health insurance was tied to employment. People without employer-based health insurance went without or paid large sums to purchase it themselves in the private market.

By the early 1990s, there was another attempt to achieve a health insurance system that would provide all people with at least basic health coverage. Under President Bill Clinton, health care reform was proposed, but ultimately defeated. Not until 2009, under President Barack Obama, did the United States finally achieve universal coverage. However, the bill is not simple, administratively, as are both Medicare and Medicaid. It is not a single payer, but a multiple payer system, and the bill is still being scrutinized by all stakeholders to determine its costs and benefits.

REFERENCES

Centers for Disease Control and Prevention. (2009, January 27). *About BMI for children and teens.* Retrieved October 12, 2009, from http://www.cdc.gov/healthyweight/assessing/bmi/childrens_bmi/about_childrens_bmi.html

Centers for Disease Control and Prevention. (2010a). *About CDC's Injury Center.* Retrieved July 22, 2010, from http://cdc.gov/injury/about/index.html

Centers for Disease Control and Prevention. (2010b). *Child passenger safety: Fact sheet.* Retrieved July 20, 2010, from http://www.cdc.gov/MotorVehicleSafety/Child_Passenger_Safety/CPS-Factsheet.html

Centers for Disease Control and Prevention. (2010c). *Division of nutrition, physical activity and obesity: About us.* Retrieved August 2, 2010, from http://www.cdc.gov/nccdphp/DNPAO/aboutus/index.html

Centers for Disease Control and Prevention. (2010d). *Home.* Retrieved July 20, 2010, from http://www.cdc.gov

Centers for Disease Control and Prevention. (2010e). *Motor vehicle safety.* Retrieved July 20, 2010, from http://www.cdc.gov/MotorVehicleSafety/

Centers for Disease Control and Prevention. (2010f). *Protect the ones you love.* Retrieved August 2, 2010, from http://cdc.gov/SafeChild/Road_Traffic_Injuries/

Centers for Disease Control and Prevention. (2010g). *Teen drivers: CDC activities.* Retrieved July 20, 2010, from http://www.cdc.gov/MotorVehicleSafety/Teen_Drivers/CDC_Activities.html

Centers for Disease Control and Prevention. (2010h). *Teen Drivers: Fact Sheet.* Retrieved August 2, 2010, from http://cdc.gov/MotorVehicleSafety/Teen_Drivers/teendrivers_factsheet.html

Centers for Disease Control and Prevention. (2010i). Public Health Injury Surveillance and Prevention Program: About the Program. Retrieved October 25, 2010 from http://www.cdc.gov/ncipc/profiles/core_state/about.htm

Centers for Disease Control and Prevention. (2010j). *Childhood overweight and obesity.* Retrieved October 25, 2010, from http://www.cdc.gov/obesity/childhood/index.html

Dehghan, M., Akhtar-Danesh, N., & Merchant, A. T. (2005). Childhood obesity, prevalence and prevention. *Nutrition Journal, 4*(24). Retrieved from PubMed Central (PMC1208949)

Elder, R. W., Nichols, J. L., Shults, R. A., Sleet, D. A., Barrios, L. C., Compton R., et al. (2005). Effectiveness of school-based programs for reducing drinking and driving and riding with drinking drivers: A systematic review. *American Journal of Preventive Medicine, 28,* 288–304.

Freedman, D. S., Khan, L. K., Dietz, W. H., Srinivasan, S. R., & Berenson, G. S. (2001). Relationship to coronary heart disease risk factors in adulthood: The Bogalusa heart study. *Pediatrics, 108*(3), 712–718.

Friedlander, S. L., Larkin, E. K., Rosen C. L., Palermo, T. M., & Redline, S. (2003). Decreased quality of life associated with childhood obesity. *Archives of Pediatrics & Adolescent Medicine, 157,* 1206–1211.

International Association for the Study of Obesity. (2010). Global trends in childhood overweight. Retrieved October 25, 2010, from http://www.iotf.org/database/Trendsinchildrenmaps.htm

Hu, F. B., Li T. Y., Colditz, G. A., Willet W. C., & Manson J. E. (2003). Television watching and other sedentary behaviors in relation to risk of obesity and type 2 diabetes. *Journal of American Medical Association, 289,* 1785–1791.

International Obesity Taskforce. (2009). *Childhood obesity.* Retrieved October 7, 2009, from www.iotf.org/childhoodobesity.asp

Institute of Medicine. (2004). *Childhood obesity in the United States: Facts and figures*. Retrieved September 30, 2009, from http://www.iom.edu

Keener, D., Goodman, K., Lowry, A., Zaro, S., & Kettel Khan, L. (2009). *Recommended community strategies and measurements to prevent obesity in the United States: Implementation and measurement guide*. Atlanta, GA: U.S. Department of Health and Human Services, Centers for Disease Control and Prevention.

Khan, L. K., & Bowman, B. A. (1999). Obesity: A major global public health problem. *Annual Review of Nutrition, 19*, xiii–xvii.

Kimm, S. Y., & Obarzanek, E. (2002). Childhood obesity: A new pandemic of the new millennium. *Pediatrics, 110*(5), 1003–1007.

LaFontaine, T. (2008). Physical activity: The epidemic of obesity and overweight among youth: Trends, consequences, and interventions. *American Journal of Lifestyle Medicine, 2*(1), 30–36.

Li, L., Law, C., Lo Conte, R., & Power, C. (2009). Intergenerational influences on childhood body mass index: The effect of parental body mass index trajectories. *The American Journal of Clinical Nutrition, 89*(2), 551–557.

McNeely, C., & Crosnoe R. (2008). Social status peer influence, and weight gain in adolescence: Promising directions for addressing the obesity epidemic. *Archives of Pediatrics & Adolescent Medicine, 162*, 91–92.

National Center for Health Statistics. (2010a). *About the national health and nutrition examination survey*. Retrieved August 2, 2010, from http://www.cdc.gov/nchs/nhanes/about_nhanes.htm

National Center for Health Statistics. (2010b). *Health, United States, 2009: With special feature on medical technology*. Hyattsville, MD: National Center for Health Statistics.

Ogden, C. L., Carroll, M. D., Curtin, L. R., McDowell, M. A., Tabak, C. J., & Flegal, K. M. (2006). Prevalence of overweight and obesity in the United States, 1994–2004. *The Journal of the American Medical Association, 295*(13), 1549–1555.

Robinson, T. N. (1998). Does television cause childhood obesity? *Journal of American Medical Association, 279*, 959–960.

Serdula, M. K., Ivery, D., Coates, R. J., Freedman, D. S., Williamson, D. F., & Byers, T. (1993). Do obese children become obese adults? A review of the literature. *Preventive Medicine, 22*(2), 167–177.

Simons-Morton, B., & Hartos, J., (Eds.). (2002). Reducing young driver crash risk: Proceedings of an expert conference on young drivers. *Injury Prevention, 8*(Suppl II), ii1–ii2.

Strauss, R. S. (2000). Childhood obesity and self-esteem, *Pediatrics, 105*(1), e15.

Task Force on Community Preventive Services, (2005). *The guide to community preventive services: What works to promote health*. New York: Oxford University Press.

Trevino, R. P., Fogt, D. L., Wyatt, T. J., Leal-Vasquez, L., Sosa, E., & Woods, C. (2008). Diabetes risk, low fitness, and energy insufficiency levels among children from poor families. *Journal of the American Dietetic Association*, *108*(11), 1846–1853.

Whitaker, R. C., Wright, J. A., Pepe, M. S., Seidel, K. D., & Dietz, W. H. (1997). Predicting obesity in young adulthood from childhood and parental obesity. *New England Journal of Medicine*, *337*(13), 869–873.

World Health Organization. (2010a). *Childhood overweight and obesity.* Retrieved October 26, 2010, from http://www.who.int/dietphysicalactivity/childhood/en/

World Health Organization. (2010b). *Obesity and overweight.* Retrieved October 25, 2010, from http://www.who.int/mediacentre/factsheets/fs311/en/index.html

6

Public Health System Performance

ACCOUNTABILITY AND EVIDENCE-BASED PUBLIC HEALTH

Evaluation of the public health system is increasingly important in this era of accountability and finite budgets. Like the health care system, the public health system's performance is generally evaluated on three criteria: (a) effectiveness, (b) efficiency, and (c) equity (Aday, Begley, Lairson, & Balkrishnan, 2004; Aday, Begley, Lairson, & Slater, 1993). Therefore, the overall evaluation of public health performance asks the question: How effective, efficient, and equitable is public health in achieving its mission to prevent disease, injury, disability, and premature death by "assuring conditions in which people can be healthy?" (IOM, 1988, p. 1)

Effectiveness focuses on whether the desired benefits of public health practices—programs, policies, services—are achieved. Efficiency focuses on how the benefits achieved by public health compare to the resources expended to realize them, and whether alternate practices would have achieved greater benefits or the same benefits using fewer resources. "Equity addresses the fairness and effectiveness of policies in minimizing population health disparities" (Aday, 2005, p. 2). The effectiveness, efficiency, and equity criteria are often complimentary. Improving effectiveness while holding resources constant increases efficiency, and those increases in efficiency may create opportunities for improved effectiveness and equity. These criteria—effectiveness, efficiency, and equity—provide a basis for evaluating the performance of the public health system, as they do for evaluating the health care system.

It is a tremendously complex undertaking to provide answers to questions about public health performance. At what level do we measure success? What indices of success do we use? Public health performance may be assessed at the micro level—for single groups, organizations, communities, and geographically specific populations—or at the macro level—for counties, regions, states, and nations. For example, at the micro level, we may be interested in the success rate of one public health program to prevent smoking in a single group within a community. At the macro level, we may want to know how one state compares to another in rates of smoking.

197

Performance indicators may be specific to a single public health service or general, reflecting the performance of numerous services and disease-specific initiatives. For example, we may evaluate food inspection services in a county based on rates of foodborne illnesses in that county, or we may assess the overall effectiveness of all public health services in the county based on a general measure of health status such as premature death rates. We can evaluate public health performance against several types of referents. We can use a "gold standard" to determine whether we have achieved the recognized "best" possible performance, if there is a "gold standard." We can use our own previous performance as a "benchmark" to determine whether we have improved over time. We can use a "benchmark" from another entity to determine whether we are doing as well as or better than an appropriate referent—organization, community, population, region, state, or nation.

The movement to evaluate public health performance, systematically, has resulted in the need to substantiate what works and what does not work in public health practice—*evidence-based public health*—based on scientifically valid empirical research. We explicitly seek to base our initiatives, programs, and policies aimed at preventing disease, injury, disability, and premature death in populations on knowledge that has resulted from sound research about the effectiveness, efficiency, and equity of public health practices. As Kohatsu and his colleagues write, "Decisions and policies in public health are frequently driven by crises, political concerns, and public opinion. A number of researchers, however, are proposing a more evidence-based approach to public health, based on the advances of evidence-based medicine" (Kohatsu, Robinson, & Torner, 2004, p. 417).

The logic of evidence based practice identifies a cyclic relation between evaluation, evidence, practice, and further evaluation. It is based on the premise that evaluations determine whether anticipated intervention effects occur in practice, and identify unanticipated effects. The reports of such evaluations are a valuable source of evidence to maximize the benefits, and reduce the harms, of public health policy and practice. The evidence can also inform evaluation planning, and thus improve the quality and relevance new research. (Rychetnik, Hawe, Waters, Barratt, & Frommer, 2004, p. 541)

Table 6.1 compares three well-known definitions of evidence-based public health. Taken together, we see that the essence of *evidence-based public health* is the development of information, using scientific principles, which can inform public health practice so that it is effective, efficient, and equitable.

TABLE 6.1   Three Definitions of Evidence-Based Public Health

Definition 1[a]	Definition 2[b]	Definition 3[c]
EBPH is the conscientious, explicit, and judicious use of current best evidence in making decisions about the care of communities and populations in the domain of health protection, disease prevention, health maintenance and improvement (health promotion).	EBPH is the development, implementation, and evaluation of effective programs and policies in public health through application of principles of scientific reasoning, including systematic uses of data and information systems and appropriate use of program-planning models.	EBPH is the process of integrating science-based interventions with community preferences to improve the health of populations.

Note: EBPH = evidence-based public health. Source: Kohatsu, Robinson, & Torner, 2004.
[a] Jenicek, 1997; [b] Brownson, Gurney, & Land, 1999; Brownson, Baker, Leet, & Gillespie, 2003; [c] Kohatsu, Robinson, & Torner, 2004.

The importance of community preferences is explicitly noted in the most recent definition (Kohatsu, Robinson, & Torner 2004), because this issue has considerable bearing on the effectiveness of public health practices, as will be discussed later in this chapter.

Evidence-based public health is an activity with direct parallels to evidence-based medicine. The goals and general methods are the same, although some of the specifics differ because of the differences between medicine and public health. As some authors have noted, public health is a broader, more diverse field, and therefore a wider range of scientific approaches is needed to gather information for practice improvement. Kohatsu et al. (2004) have identified differences between evidence-based medicine and evidence-based public health, which are summarized in Table 6.2.

In general, performance evaluation takes place at two levels: (a) the individual program, policy, or service level; or (b) the population level using population mortality and morbidity measures, where these global measures are used to assess macro-level performance. Evidence-based public health usually refers to the program, policy, or service level.

Evaluations at the level of specific programs, services, or policies have identified goals that are targeted at defined populations. Therefore, measures of effectiveness, that is, measures that indicate whether the desired or intended result was brought about, are population and program specific. The basic components of any evaluation—program or system—are structure, process, and outcomes. When assessing a program, service, or policy, structure refers to the resources available to the public health program including organization and financing; the characteristics of the populations

TABLE 6.2   A Comparison of Processes: Evidence-Based Medicine Versus Evidence-Based Public Health

Step	Evidence-Based Medicine[a]	Evidence-Based Public Health[b]
1. State the scientific question of interest	Convert the need for information (about prevention, diagnosis, prognosis, therapy, causation) into an answerable question.	Develop an initial statement of the issue.
2. Identify the relevant evidence	Track down the best evidence to answer that question.	Search the scientific literature and organize information.
3. Determine what information is relevant to answering the scientific question of interest	Critically appraise that evidence for its validity (closeness to the truth), impact (size of the effect), and applicability (usefulness in one's clinical practice).	Quantify the issue using sources of existing data.
4. Determine the best course of action considering the patient or population.	Integrate the critical appraisal with one's clinical expertise and with the patient's unique biology, values, and circumstances.	Develop and prioritize program options; develop an action plan and implement interventions.
5. Evaluate process and outcome.	Evaluate one's effectiveness and efficiency in executing Steps 1 to 4 and seek ways to improve both for the next time.	Evaluate the program or policy.

Source: Kohatsu, Robinson, & Torner, 2004.
[a] Sackett Strauss, Richardson, Rosenberg, & Haynes, 2000; [b] Brownson, Gurney, & Land, 1999; Brownson, Baker, Leet, & Gillespie, 2003.

targeted by the program, service, or policy; and the physical, social, and economic environments in which the program occurs. Process refers to the implementation of the public health program, service, or policy. Outcomes refer to the expected results of implementation. Program-specific outcomes usually consist of short-term goals, such as a change in knowledge and attitudes; longer term goals, such as change in behavior; and impact, such as change in health status. Each of these goals would be specific to the program and the targeted population.

Issel (2009) provides an excellent description of the types of program evaluations. The two most useful concepts are process and outcomes evaluations. "Process evaluations focus on the degree to which the program has been implemented as planned and on the quality of the program implementation. Process evaluations are known by a variety of terms, such as monitoring evaluations, depending on their focus and characteristics" (p. 19). Outcome evaluations, often used interchangeably with impact evaluations, focus on whether the goals of the program, service, or policy have been achieved and whether the changes desired can be attributed to the program (Issel, 2009).

As an example, a project in a local school used theater to reduce intolerance among 10th graders. The theater production was developed by a group of young actors using the results of focus groups with 10th-grade students. The focus groups identified concerns of the student body. The theater production contained skits based on the personal experiences of students, increasing the relevance of the production to the audience. The short-term goals of the program—by the end of the performance—were to increase knowledge about what constitutes intolerance and how intolerance is perceived by both the victim and perpetrator. The longer term goal—during the remainder of the school year—was to increase discussions among students about tolerance issues. The desired impact of the program was a decrease in the number of incidences of intolerance reported in high school.

Population Level Outcomes[1]

Population level indicators are often the measure of impact of a program, service, or policy. These include population mortality and morbidity rates. Historically, population health indicators have been age-adjusted death rates, disease-specific death rates, life expectancy, time lost to premature death, and infant mortality rate (IMR). The United Nations International Children's Emergency Fund's (UNICEF) definition of IMR is the probability of dying between birth and exactly 1 year of age (UNICEF, 2010). This rate is expressed per 1,000 live births per year. IMR is an important measure that indicates the well-being of infants, children, and pregnant women, as it is associated with maternal health, quality and access to care, and public health in a given population. Life expectancy is defined by the World Health Organization (WHO) as the number of years of life that can be expected on average in a given population.

By using the life expectancy within that population, the time lost to premature death, also called years of potential life lost or YPLL, can be calculated. YPLL indicates that death occurred at an age less than what would be expected, and the more premature a death, the greater the loss of life (WHO, 2006a). A more recent concept of population health takes into

---

[1] Section taken from Jonas, S., Goldsteen, R. L., & Goldsteen, K. (2007). *An introduction to the U.S. health care system* (6th ed.). New York, NY: Springer Publishing.

account quality of life. Healthy life expectancy (HALE) at birth is defined by WHO as the "average number of years that a person can expect to live in 'full health' by taking into account years lived in less than full health due to disease and/or injury" (WHO, 2006a). HALE is a measure that "combines length and quality of life into a single estimate that indicates years that can be expected in a specified state of health" (Kindig, 1997, p. 45). Other health-adjusted life expectancy measures are quality-adjusted life years (QALY), which emphasizes the individual's perceived health status as the indicator of quality of life; disability-adjusted life years (DALY), which combines mortality and disability measures; and years of healthy life (YHL), which combines perceived health and disability activity limitation measures from the National Health Interview Survey (Kindig, 1997).

Mortality rate is the number of deaths in a given population per year (WHO, 2006a). The age-adjusted mortality rate takes into account the population's age distribution when calculating mortality rate. Using a statistical method that "standardizes" the target population to a reference population, this measure is commonly used when comparing mortality rates across different populations.

Sources of Evidence-Based Public Health

The following sites provide links to scientific studies and published reports that provide practical guidance to local health departments, health care providers, community leaders, employers, and others on the effectiveness of programs, services, and policies on achieving public health goals:

Agency for Healthcare Research and Quality
- Electronic Preventive Services Selector
- Offers a practical tool to assist clinicians identify appropriate preventive, screening, and counseling services for patients (www.ahrq.gov).

Association of State and Territorial Health Officials
- Presents evidence-based public health highlights initiatives and research focused on increasing the evidence base supporting public healthy interventions (www.astho.org).

Centers for Disease Control and Prevention
- Guide to Community Preventive Services
- Provides a summary of effective community interventions that promote health and prevent disease. The *Guide* is a valuable source of systematic

reviews and evidence-based recommendations for public health practice. In addition, the Task Force on Community Preventive Services and Centers for Disease Control and Prevention, who sponsor the *Guide*, have developed methods that may be used to evaluate the impact of evidence-based public health interventions (www.cdc.gov).

The Cochrane Collaboration

■ Contains a library of systematic reviews of the effects of health care interventions. The Collaboration's Health Promotion and Public Health Field (HPPHF) is aimed at increasing the quality and quantity of systematic reviews that can be used to provide evidence to answer practical, public health questions (www.cochrane.org).

E-Roadmap to Evidence-Based Public Health Practice

■ Comprehensive database of evidence-based public health practice programs and a learning tutorial that teach skills to identify and use effective programs (http://www.healthsolutions.org).

ExpectMore.gov

■ ExpectMore.gov (developed by the U.S. Office of Management and Budget and Federal Agencies) is an assessment of the performance of every federal program (expectmore.gov).

National Association of County and City Health Officials

■ National Association of County and City Health Officials (NACCHO) Model Practices Database
■ Has a searchable database of local health agency model practices, divided into community, environmental, and public health categories (www.naccho.org).

New York State Department of Health

■ Community Health Assessment Clearinghouse links to evidence-based practice resources, examples of strong community health assessments, data, and describes the 10-step process for conducting community health assessments (www.health.state.ny.us/).

PUBLIC HEALTH SYSTEM IMPROVEMENT

As discussed previously, there are two basic types of evaluation: process and outcomes evaluation. This is true of systems as well as programs, services,

204 Introduction to Public Health

and policies. In this section on public health system performance, we turn first to process improvement initiatives.

Accreditation and Credentialing

Desired outcomes result from well-thought out, well-executed processes. This is true of the public health system, as it is of any other system. Therefore, the performance of the public health system depends first on the quality and commitment of the workforce; and second, on the quality of policies, services, and programs in public health organizations at every level—local, state, and federal; and third, on the quality of data that are available to assess performance. There are several initiatives intended to ensure the quality of these three aspects of the public health system. The quality of the workforce is addressed by the accreditation of public health programs and schools by the Council on Education for Public Health (CEPH); the core competencies project developed by the Public Health Foundation's (PHF) Council on Linkages Between Academia and Public Health Practice; and the certification of individual public health professionals by the National Board of Public Health Examiners (NBPHE). The quality of policies, services, and programs in public health organizations is addressed by the accreditation of state and local public health departments by the Public Health Accreditation Board (PHAB). Data that are needed to assess and improve public health system performance are continually being developed, and some important sources of evidence-based public health are listed earlier in this chapter (under "Sources of Evidence-Based Public Health"). One that we will discuss later is the report card initiative.

The organizations involved in improving public health performance are private, nonprofit entities, supported by members and organizations, chief among them are the American Public Health Association, the Association of Schools of Public Health (ASPH), and the Association for Prevention Teaching and Research. The Association of State and Territorial Health Officials, the National Association of County and City Health Officials, the National Association of Local Boards of Health, and the National Indian Health Board have also been heavily involved with accreditation of health departments. Several private foundations have been committed to improving public health performance through these initiatives including the Robert Wood Johnson Foundation, the American Legacy Foundation, the Foundation to Advance Public Health through Certification, and the Josiah Macy, Jr. Foundation. Each certification—individual, educational program, and public health organization—is voluntary at this time, although CEPH accreditation confers many benefits on schools and programs of public health and their graduates.

Council on Education for Public Health

The CEPH is one of the oldest of the initiatives. CEPH is "an independent agency recognized by the U.S. Department of Education to accredit schools of public health and certain public health programs offered in settings other than schools of public health" (CEPH, 2010, para. 1). These schools and programs prepare students for entry into careers in public health. The primary professional degree is the Master of Public Health (MPH), but other masters and doctoral degrees are offered as well. The goal of the Council is "to enhance health in human populations through organized community effort" (CEPH, 2010, para. 2).

The Council's focus is the improvement of health through the assurance of professional personnel who are able to identify, prevent and solve community health problems. The Council's objectives are:

1. to promote quality in public health education through a continuing process of self-evaluation by the schools and programs that seek accreditation;
2. to assure the public that institutions offering graduate instruction in public health have been evaluated and judged to meet standards essential for the conduct of such educational programs; and
3. to encourage—through periodic review, consultation, research, publications, and other means—improvements in the quality of education for public health. (CEPH, 2010, para. 3)

CEPH evaluates the curriculum of programs and schools of public health based on the competencies that were developed by the ASPH, which contain five core areas (biostatistics, environmental health sciences, epidemiology, health policy and management, social and behavioral sciences) and seven crosscutting areas (communications and informatics, diversity and cultural proficiency, leadership, professionalism and ethics, program planning and assessment, public health biology, and systems thinking [ASPH, 2010]).

As of the writing of this book, there were 44 accredited schools of public health and 82 accredited programs in public health, mostly in the United States (CEPH, 2010).

Core Competencies for Public Health Professionals Project

The PHF has developed a set of core competencies for public health professionals through its Council on Linkages Between Academia and Public Health Practice. The most recent version of the core competencies has three tiers, which differentiate the skills needed by entry-level individuals, individuals with management and/or supervisory responsibilities, and senior level managers and/or leaders of public health organizations. There are seven skill domains within the core competencies: analytical/assessment; policy development/program planning; communication; cultural competency; community dimensions of practice; public health sciences; financial planning and management. Core competencies are used by educational programs to build their curriculum and by public health organizations to identify their workforce needs (PHF, 2010).

National Board of Public Health Examiners

The NBPHE was established in 2005 as an independent organization to make certain that students and graduates from CEPH-accredited schools and programs of public health have mastered the knowledge and skills required by contemporary public health. To this end, the NBPHE has administered the Certified in Public Health (CPH) exam each year, beginning in 2009. In addition to developing, administering, and scoring the exam, the NBPHE prepares students to take the exam through study guides and study sessions. The CPH exam is another method of ensuring the quality of the public health workforce.

The goals of credentialing are to:

- Increase recognition of the public health professions
- Raise the visibility of public health
- Set standards of knowledge and skills in public health
- Foster environment of a professional community
- Encourage life-long learning (NBPHE, 2010, para. 2)

To be eligible for the CPH exam, applicants must have a graduate level degree from a CEPH-accredited school or program of public health. CPH professionals are required to obtain 50 hours of continuing education every 2 years, and they will be required to complete a reassessment every 10 years. The CPH exam covers the core areas of knowledge in CEPH-accredited schools and programs and is based on the Masters of Public

Health competencies. There were 558 persons in the Charter Class of Certified in Public Health Examinees (NBPHE, 2010).

Public Health Accreditation Board

The newest accrediting body for public health is the PHAB, whose goal is "to improve and protect the health of every community by advancing the quality and performance of public health departments" (PHAB, 2010, para. 1). State and local health departments are the target for this accreditation initiative:

> In order to improve the health of the public, the Public Health Accreditation Board (PHAB) is developing a national voluntary accreditation program for state, local, territorial and tribal public health departments. The goal of the accreditation program is to improve and protect the health of every community by advancing the quality and performance of public health departments. (PHAB, 2010, para. 1)

The initiative to accredit local health departments originated with the groundbreaking report, *The Future of Public Health* (Institute of Medicine [IOM], 1988), which was sponsored by the IOM. The report galvanized public health with a study that had been in the making for 10 years after the IOM assessment that there was a "deplorable lack of reliability, even availability, of an identifiable local component of the public health system in many parts of the country and an unexplainable variability in configuration and performance in the rest of the country" (Tilson, 2008, p. xv). Tilson has written an excellent summary of the history of public health accreditation, part of which is repeated in the following boxed text:

The IOM committee reframed the mission of public health as "fulfilling society's interest in assuring conditions in which people can be healthy" (8, p. 7). And the committee created a new conceptual framework with which to comprehend the scope of public health's activities as core functions at all government levels: assessment, policy development, and assurance. Into that landmark IOM report a prior thread was woven to strengthen the fabric. *The Model Standards for Community Preventive Health Services* (1) were recognized as providing necessary materials with which to weave this new cloth.

These standards, in turn, had undergone a ten-year development process under the leadership of the Centers for Disease and Prevention (CDC). They were initiated at CDC in response to the public health delivery system's failure in the United States to respond adequately or coherently to the substantial challenges in a short-notice nationwide immunization initiative against swine influenza in 1976. For each of the major content areas of public health practice, indicators recognizable and countable in any local community were identified through a consensus process deriving from the same leadership organizations now working together on accreditation. As model standards, the proposal outlined the challenges to the local community using an open-ended, fill-in-the-blanks approach to modeling: By 19xx, the rate of problem Y will not exceed (or will be reduced to) Z. In association with the Healthy People 2000 undertaking, an effort at depicting benchmarks, the project developed either national averages or synthetic composite metrics from multiple reporting jurisdictions about each of the objectives in the *Model Standards*, now still part of the Healthy People publications. . . . The IOM and many other advocates saw that accreditation could be done in such a way as to recognize local unique situations but still achieve the dual purposes of accountability and continuous process improvement. They based this position on what they observed to be a breakthrough concept, the National Public Health System Performance Standards, which "provide a way to conceptualize the system as the unit of accreditation and, from there, to evaluate the role of the agencies in facilitating the work of the system" (Tilson, 2008, p. xvi).

The current accreditation program administered by the PHAB has three core components: domains, standards, and measurements. Domains are the competencies and broad areas of responsibility for a health department and are based on the 10 essential public health services, National Public Health Performance Standards System (NPHPSS), and the NACCHO Operational Definition, and others. "Standards are expected levels of performance that reflect a specific responsibility within a domain. For example, the NPHPSP (local level) has 32 model standards for its 10 domains. A measure consists of a metric to assess the extent to which a standard is met. Each standard can have one or more measures that reflect a specific level of performance achievement and skill competency" (Bialek, Duffy, & Moran, 2009, p. 54).

Eligible applicants for PHAB accreditation are "any government entity with primary legal responsibility for public health in a state, territory, and tribe or at the local level" (PHAB, 2010). The domains are:

- Monitor health status and understand health issues;
- Protect people from health problems and health hazards;
- Give people information they need to make health choices;
- Engage the community to identify and solve health problems;
- Develop public health policies and plans;
- Enforce public health laws and regulations;
- Help people receive health services;
- Maintain a competent public health workforce;
- Use continuous quality improvement tools to evaluate and improve the quality of programs and interventions;
- Contribute to and apply the evidence base of public health; and
- Govern and manage health department resources (including financial and human resources, facilities and information systems).

Report Card Initiatives

The report card initiatives can be viewed as outcomes evaluations of the public health system as a whole. They collect, organize, and present information about the outcomes that are central to the public health system: population health status, morbidity, and mortality. These indicators are used in macro-level performance evaluations of such areas as cities, counties, regions, states, and nations. We assume the impact of public health care on these rates even though we are not directly measuring exposure to any specific public health service, program, or initiative among the population considered. If, for example, an infectious disease-specific mortality rate is higher in one region than another, we assume that the public health system (and health care system) has not been optimal in the region with the higher mortality rate.

The initiatives discussed here are Healthy People, state report cards, and America's Health Rankings.

Healthy People

Healthy People, the health promotion and disease prevention agenda for the United States, sets health objectives for the nation, monitors progress toward achieving those objectives, and issues regular reports on the results. Healthy People has been a highly influential initiative for assessing the health of the nation and, by implication, the performance of the public health system. The Healthy People initiative acknowledges that even though the agenda is national, the improvements will come through local actions, which will then affect the state, regional, and national outcomes reports.

The history of Healthy People spans 3 decades (CDC, 2010a; CDC, 2010b). The initiative is an outgrowth of *Healthy People: The Surgeon General's Report on Health Promotion and Disease Prevention* (Office of the Assistant Secretary for Health and Surgeon General, 1979), a document presenting quantitative goals to reduce preventable death and injury by 1990. In 1980, the U.S. Public Health Service released a companion report, which contained specific, quantifiable objectives to achieve the Healthy People goals. Since then, the U.S. Department of Health and Human Services (DHHS) has updated these national health promotion and disease prevention goals and objectives each decade in Healthy People 2000 (IOM, 1990) and Healthy People 2010 (DHHS, 2000).

The goals of the first Healthy People initiative were to reduce mortality among four age groups—infants, children, adolescents and young adults, and adults—and increase independence among older adults. There were 15 priority areas and 226 objectives. Healthy People 2000 had three overarching goals: to increase years of healthy life, reduce disparities in health among different population groups, and achieve access to preventive health services. There were 22 priority areas, with 319 supporting objectives. Healthy People 2010 had two overarching goals: to increase quality and years of healthy life and to eliminate health disparities, which served to guide the development of objectives that would be used to measure progress. There were 28 focus areas (changed from priority areas) and 467 objectives.

The process of selecting priority/focus areas for Healthy People has become more participatory over time.

> The process for creating objectives evolved from one that was largely expert-driven with opportunities for feedback from the public (for the 1990 Health Objectives), to one that emphasized public engagement, feedback, and participation throughout the development process (for Healthy People 2010). Emphasis on public participation has continued in the two-phased process for developing Healthy People 2020. (DHHS, 2010, para. 3)

The CDC's National Center for Health Statistics (NCHS) is responsible for monitoring Healthy People objectives using its own and other data sources. As a result, there is a great deal of dependence on the data collected at state and local levels from government and nongovernment organizations. The NCHS makes data available through DATA2010, an interactive database system accessible through the NCHS Web site, and the CDC WONDER system. The online *Tracking Healthy People 2010* publication informs that effort. This report includes technical information on general data issues and major data sources, detailed definitions for each objective, and additional resources (DHHS, 2010).

Healthy People has become a strategic management tool—for the federal government, states, communities, and many private sector partners:

> To date, 47 States, the District of Columbia, and Guam have developed their own Healthy People plans. Most states have emulated national objectives, but virtually all have tailored them to their specific needs. A 1993 National Association of County and City Health Officials survey showed that 70 percent of local health departments use Healthy People 2000 objectives. Within the Federal Government, Healthy People provides a framework for measuring performance in the Government Performance and Results Act. Success is measured by positive changes in health status or reductions in risk factors, as well as improved provision of services. Progress reviews are conducted periodically on each of the 22 priority areas and on population groups, including women, adolescents, people with disabilities, and racial/ethnic groups. Healthy People objectives have been specified by Congress as the metric for measuring the progress of the Indian Health Service, the Maternal and Child Health Block Grant, and the Preventive Health and Health Services Block Grant. Ongoing involvement is ensured through the *Healthy People Consortium*—an alliance of 350 national membership organizations and 300 state health, mental health, substance abuse, and environmental agencies. (Healthy People 2000, 2010)

As with all initiatives, Healthy People has encountered challenges and been the target of criticisms. Criticisms include its printed format that constrains usability; the extensive list of objectives that are hard to manage; a disease-specific approach to organizing objectives that has not encouraged cross-cutting collaboration around risk factors; lack of transparency about target-setting methods for specific objectives; and lack of data to assess progress.

Several criticisms about Healthy People seem inappropriate, including lack of progress or slow progress in achieving objective targets; inadequate guidance on how to achieve the objectives; and lack of guidance to users in setting priorities. As a report card system, it can be argued that the Healthy People initiative is not responsible for achieving the targets. Rather, the public health system, as a whole, is accountable for progress toward Healthy People objectives.

Table 6.3 contains summary information about the nation's progress toward achieving Healthy People objectives. There was a greater success in achieving 1990 objectives than those in 2000 or 2010 (midcourse)—32%, 21%, and 6% achieved, respectively. Also note that 40% of the 2010 objectives could not be assessed, because we lack tracking data.

Healthy People has raised awareness—as all good report cards do—about the public health problems that we have, the progress that we have made toward solving them, and the problems that remain unsolved, and therefore, in need of continued attention and action. Healthy People results show, especially, that we have not been able to eliminate health

TABLE 6.3   Most Recent Data on Achievement of Past Healthy People Objectives

Most Recent Data Source	Number of Objectives/ Targets	Achieved Target	Progressed Toward Target	Showed No Progress or Regressed from Target	Data Unavailable
1990 Health objectives *(Final review)* NCHS, 1992	226 objectives, 266 targets[a]	32%	34%	11%	23%
Healthy People 2000[b] *(Final review)* NCHS, 2001	319	21%	41%	17%	10%
Healthy People 2010 *(Midcourse review)* DHHS, 2006[c]	467	6%	30%	16%	40%[d]

Note: NCHS = National Center for Health Statistics; DHHS = U.S. Department of Health and Human Services.
[a]All percentages for the 1990 Health objectives reflect attainment of the 266 measured *targets*.
[b]Percentages for Healthy People 2000 objectives do not add up to 100% in this table because 11% of objectives (35) that showed mixed progress have been excluded.
[c]Percentages for Healthy People 2010 objectives do not add up to 100% in this table because 12% of objectives (57 out of 467) showed mixed progress have been excluded.
[d]This percentage includes 28 objectives that were deleted, as well as 158 objectives that could not be assessed because of a lack of tracking data.
Source: DHHS, 2010

disparities between white and minority populations at the community level (DHHS, 2010). Although health care has been proposed as the solution to health disparities, the ecological orientation of public health tells us that health care alone will not eliminate them. "Health disparities, however, are multidimensional, complicated issues that cannot be addressed through the provision of health care alone. Health disparities are rooted in fundamental social structure inequalities" (Aday, 2005, p. 241).

State Report Cards

Many states and local health departments provide report cards on their progress and a report of the status in that geographical area. An example is New York State, which has report cards for the state and its counties. The Community Health Assessment Clearinghouse is a "one-stop" resource for community health planners, practitioners, and policy developers.

Data
- New York Community Health Data Set (updated July 2009)
- County Health Assessment Indicators (CHAI; updated July 2009)
- County Health Indicators by Race/Ethnicity (CHIRE; New May 2010)
- County Health Indicator Profiles (updated July 2009)
- Data for states including New York
- National public health data sets

How-To Guide
- New York State Community Health Assessment Guidance Documents
- 10-step assessment process with worksheets

Examples
- U.S. sources of evidence-based public health
- International sources of evidence-based public health
- Promising Practices Resources
- Community health assessments and report cards

See New York State Department of Health (NYS DOH) Web site for additional information at http://www.health.state.ny.us/statistics/chac/index.htm

America's Health Rankings

America's Health Rankings™ is a 20-year-old report card initiative that ranks each state on health outcomes and health determinants for the purpose of helping localities, counties, states and regions make decisions about how to improve population health.

> The 22 measures that comprise America's Health Rankings™ are of two types—health determinants and health outcomes. Health determinants represent those actions that can affect the future health of the population, whereas health outcomes represent the result of what has already occurred, either through death or missed days due to illness. For a state to improve the health of its population, efforts must focus on changing the determinants of health. If a state is significantly better in its ranking for health determinants than its ranking for health outcomes, it will be more likely to improve its overall health ranking in the future. Conversely, if a state is worse in its ranking for health determinants than its ranking for health outcomes, its overall health ranking will be more *likely to decline over time* [emphasis added]. (America's Health Rankings, 2010, para. 2)

The initiative is a joint project of the United Health Foundation, the American Public Health Association, and Partnership for Prevention.

The model used by America's Health Rankings is reproduced in Figure 6.1. It is an ecological model that includes behaviors, policy, health care, and the community and other environments. Table 6.4 contains the measures that are included in each state's scores.

As an example, Table 6.5 contains information from America's Health Rankings for 2009. The top five–and bottom five–ranked states on premature death are listed, along with their rankings on other measures including socioeconomic indicators, health behaviors, medical care, and public health funding. There is a general tendency for the states to be similarly ranked on premature death and other indicators. With a few exceptions, the top 5 are

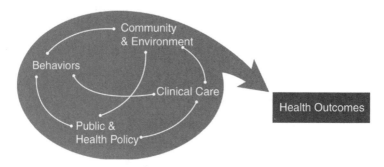

FIGURE 6.1 Components of Health. *Source:* America's Health Rankings, 2009

TABLE 6.4   American's Health Rankings, Core Measures

Behavior	Clinical Care
Prevalence of smoking	Prenatal care
Prevalence of binge drinking	Primary care physicians
Prevalence of obesity	Preventable hospitalizations
High school graduation	**Outcomes**
Community and Environment	Poor mental health days
Violent crime	Poor physical health days
Occupational fatalities	Geographic disparity
Infectious disease	Infant mortality
Children in poverty	Cardiovascular deaths
Air pollution	Cancer deaths
Public and Health Policies	Premature death
Lack of health insurance	
Public health funding	
Immunization coverage	

Source: America's Health Rankings, 2010

TABLE 6.5   Five Highest and Five Lowest Ranked States on Premature Death, With Rankings on Selected Health Determinants

Premature Death	Per Capital Income	Children in Poverty	Teen Birth Rate	Physical Activity	Obesity	Diabetes	Uninsured	Preventable Hospital Stays	Public Health Funding
Top 5 States									
1. Minnesota	10	18	10	1	13	1	3	9	46
2. New Hampshire	9	1	1	9	11	14	10	11	35
3. Vermont	22	4	2	5	7	4	9	7	2
4. Massachusetts	3	21	3	10	2	13	1	37	6
5. Connecticut	1	6	4	12	2	8	7	18	33
Bottom 5 States									
46. South Carolina	45	33	38	37	45	44	37	26	20
47. Arkansas	47	37	47	45	41	37	40	44	30
48. Alabama	41	47	39	44	49	48	18	43	14
49. Louisiana	30	44	40	46	37	47	47	47	16
50. Mississippi	50	46	50	50	50	49	43	48	29

Source: www.americashealthrankings.org/measure/2009/List All/Overall, America's Health Rankings, http://www.americashealthrankings.org. Accessed July 2010.

ranked higher than 15 and the bottom 5 are ranked lower than 35. Public health funding is the least associated with premature death, however.

Another table demonstrates the variation within states (see Table 6.6). Information about the county-level indicators was obtained from the Population Health Institute at the University of Wisconsin (2010). States ranked high by America's Health Rankings on overall health such as Vermont, Massachusetts, and New Hampshire have counties that are doing poorly. Likewise, counties that are poorly ranked, such as Mississippi, Alabama, and Louisiana have some counties that are doing well. These findings point to the importance of community-based efforts to improve health in the nation and to the disparities that exist between populations and regions.

Effectiveness and Equity of Public Health System

In the following section, we develop an informal report card for the U.S. public health system, by comparing population-level indicators across countries and within subgroups of the United States. Although these indicators are not specific to any one public health program, service, or policy, we assume the overall impact of the public health system on two of the performance criteria—effectiveness and equity—is reflected in these measures.

Life Expectancy and Age-Adjusted Mortality

As an example of how population level outcomes are used to assess public health performance, consider the case of life expectancy and age-adjusted mortality rates. Life expectancy can be used as an assessment measure in at least two ways. First, we can compare the life expectancy in one society to life expectancy in another. Second, we can compare life expectancies among subgroups within one society. In the first case, life expectancy rates indicate that the United States has a problem with public health effectiveness. In the second case, life expectancy rates indicate that the United States has a problem with equity.

First, we consider life expectancy in the United States compared to other nations. In 2004, WHO comparisons of 13 peer countries indicated that the United States ranked 10th out of 13 in life expectancy at birth for males, and 12th out of 13 in life expectancy at birth for females (WHO, 2006b). These countries are Australia, Belgium, Canada, Denmark, Finland, France, Germany, Japan, The Netherlands, Spain, Sweden, the United Kingdom, and the United States. Next, we examine life expectancy and age-adjusted

TABLE 6.6   Five Highest and Five Lowest Ranked States on Premature Death, with Selected Health Determinants by County

Selected Counties Ranked on Overall Health	Poor or Fair Health	Adult Obesity	College Degrees	Children in Poverty	Single-Parent Households	Uninsured Adults
Two Highest and Two Lowest Ranked Counties on Selected Indicators						
1. Vermont						
Chittenden	8%	19%	45%	8%	9%	12%
Addison	10%	21%	30%	10%	8%	13%
Orange	12%	26%	30%	14%	8%	15%
Essex	17%	25%	15%	21%	9%	16%
3. Massachusetts						
Nantucket	7%	20%	42%	5%	7%	20%
Norfolk	9%	19%	47%	6%	6%	10%
Hampden	15%	26%	24%	25%	12%	12%
Suffolk	17%	21%	37%	28%	11%	15%
5. New Hampshire						
Grafton	10%	23%	34%	10%	8%	14%
Rockingham	10%	23%	36%	6%	7%	10%
Sullivan	12%	27%	25%	12%	10%	13%
Coos	17%	27%	17%	17%	9%	12%
47. Louisiana						
St. Tammany	14%	26%	30%	15%	9%	23%
Lafayette	16%	25%	28%	22%	12%	22%
Madison	21%	33%	13%	49%	16%	14%
East Carroll	20%	34%	14%	56%	18%	12%
48. Alabama						
Shelby	11%	28%	39%	9%	7%	13%
Baldwin	13%	25%	26%	15%	9%	21%
Greene	20%	44%	12%	44%	16%	15%
Lowndes	N/A	40%	12%	43%	15%	15%
50. Mississippi						
DeSoto	16%	32%	20%	11%	11%	20%
Rankin	17%	29%	28%	14%	10%	19%
Tallahatchie	37%	36%	12%	40%	16%	16%
Holmes	25%	42%	12%	51%	22%	13%

Source: Population Health Institute, 2010.
N/A = Not available

mortality among subgroups within the United States. There are significant differences between population subgroups (Adler et al., 1993; IOM, 2003; Pappas, Queen, Hadden, & Fisher, 1993). In 2002, the projected life expectancy at birth for U.S. residents was 77.3 years (U.S. Census Bureau, 2005, Table 96). For men, it was 74.5 years; for women, 79.9 years. These numbers were all up from those observed in 1990, respectively, 75.4, 71.8, and 78.8. In 2002, the age-adjusted death rate was 8.5 per 1,000 population: 10.1 for males and 7.2 for females (U.S. Census Bureau, Table 99). (Age adjustment statistically accounts for the fact that life expectancy from birth is shorter for males than for females.) Again, this was an improvement over 1990 when the age-adjusted death rate was 9.4 per 1,000 population, 12.0 for males and 7.5 for females. In 2002, there was a marked difference in life expectancy at birth by race: 75.1 for White males and 68.8 for African American males (U.S. Census Bureau, Table 98). Similarly, White females had a life expectancy at birth of 80.3 compared to 75.6 for African American females. The age-adjusted death rate for White males in 2002 was 9.9 per 1,000 population, and for African American males it was 13.4 (U.S. Census Bureau, Table 99). White females had an age-adjusted mortality rate of 7.0 compared to that of African American females with 9.0. The difference in life expectancy and mortality between Whites and African Americans is thought, in part, to reflect differences in the standard of living, as well as access to health services (Geiger, 1996; IOM, 2003; Schwartz, Kofie, Rivo, & Tuckson, 1990).

Quality of Life-Adjusted Measure

The WHO (2006b) comparisons of the United States to 12 peer countries indicate, once again, that the U.S. population is not as healthy as we would expect, again indicating a problem with effectiveness. In 2002, HALE at birth for males was 67.2 years in the United States, the lowest ranked country of the 13. Japan was ranked 1 (72.3 years). For HALE at birth for females, the United States was ranked 12th out of 13 in 2002. In 2002, the age standardized DALY per 100,000 population for all causes of death was higher in the United States than in any of its 12 peer countries (12,781/100,000 population). The next highest DALY was 10,878/100,000 population in Belgium.

Infant, Neonatal, and Maternal Mortality

Comparison of IMRs in the United States to the same 13 peer countries also indicates a problem of public health effectiveness and equity in the United

States. In 2004, the U.S. IMR was 6.0 per 1,000 live births (WHO, 2006b). Although this rate is low, it is the highest of the 13 peer countries. In 2000, neonatal mortality was highest in the United States (5 per 1,000 live births), compared to its peer countries, and maternal mortality was third highest (14 maternal deaths per 100,000 live births). The subgroup comparison of infant mortality within the United States also indicates problems. The difference in the IMR in the United States between Whites and African Americans is striking. In 2002, the IMR was 5.8 for Whites and 13.8 for African Americans (U.S. Census Bureau, 2005, Table 105). The African American IMR has been at least double that for Whites since 1915, when the rate was first recorded as 99.9 per thousand overall (Grove & Hetzel, 1968).

Summary

Performance of the public health system can be evaluated at the micro level of programs, policies, and services that are targeted at defined populations, and it can be evaluated at the system level using population health indicators such as IMR, life expectancy, and premature death rate for geographic locales and subpopulations. The criteria for evaluating the public health system, as a whole, as well as its component programs, policies, and services are effectiveness, equity, and efficiency. There is strong evidence from the report card initiatives that the effectiveness and equity of the system are not satisfactory, and therefore, the efficiency of the system cannot be acceptable either.

REFERENCES

Aday, L. A. (Ed.). (2005). *Reinventing public health: Policies and practices for a healthy nation*. San Francisco: Jossey-Bass.

Aday, L. A., Begley, C. E., Lairson, D. R., & Balkrishnan, R. (2004). *Evaluating the healthcare system: Effectiveness, efficiency, and equity*. Chicago: Health Administration Press.

Aday, L. A., Begley, C. E., Lairson, D. R., & Slater, C. H. (1993). *Evaluating the medical care system: Effectiveness, efficiency, and equity*. Ann Arbor, MI: Health Administration Press.

Adler, N. E., Boyce, W. T., Chesney, M. A., Folkman, S. , Syme, S. L. (1993). *Socioeconomic inequalities in health: No easy solution*. The Journal of the American Medical Association, 269(24), 3140–3145.

America's Health Rankings. (2009). A call to action for individuals and their communities. Minnetonka, MN: United Health Foundation.

America's Health Rankings. (2010). *About the rankings*. Retrieved July 20, 2010, from http://www.americashealthrankings.org/

Association of Schools of Public Health. (2010). *Competency and learning outcomes development projects*. Retrieved July 10, 2010, from http://www.asph.org/document.cfm?page=1083

Bialek, R. G., Duffy, G. L., & Moran, J. W. (2009). *The public health quality improvement handbook*. Milwaukee, WI: American Society for Quality, Quality Press.

Brownson, R. C., Baker, E. A., Leet, T. L., & Gillespie, K. N. (2003). *Evidence-based public health*. New York: Oxford University Press.

Brownson, R. C., Gurney, J. G., & Land, G. H. (1999). Evidence-based decision making in public health. *Journal of Public Health Management and Practice, 5*, 86–97.

Centers for Disease Control and Prevention. (2010a). *Healthy people 2000*. Retrieved July 20, 2010, from http://www.cdc.gov/nchs/healthy_people/hp2000.htm

Centers for Disease Control and Prevention. (2010b). *Healthy people 2010*. Retrieved July 20, 2010, from http://www.cdc.gov/nchs/healthy_people/hp2010.htm

Council on Education for Public Health. (2010). *About CEPH*. Retrieved July 20, 2010, from http://www.ceph.org/pg_about.htm

Geiger, H. J. (1996). Race and health care—An American dilemma? *New England Journal of Medicine, 335*(11), 815–816.

Grove, R. D., & Hetzel, A. M. (1968). *Vital statistics rates in the United States: 1940–1960*. Washington, DC: U.S. Government Printing Office.

Healthy People 2000. (2010). *Healthy people 2000 fact sheet*. Retrieved July 20, 2010, from http://odphp.osophs.dhhs.gov/pubs/HP2000/hp2kfact.htm

Institute of Medicine. (1990). *Healthy people 2000: Citizens chart the course*. Washington, DC: National Academy Press.

Institute of Medicine. (2003). *Unequal treatment: Confronting racial and ethnic disparities in health care*. Washington, DC: National Academy Press.

Institute of Medicine, Committee on the Study of the Future of Public Health. (1988). *The future of public health*. Washington, DC: National Academy Press.

Issel, L. M. (2009). *Health program planning and evaluation*. Sudbury, MA: Jones and Bartlett.

Jenicek, M. (1997). *Epidemiology, evidence-based medicine, and evidence-based public health*. Journal of Epidemiology, 7, 187–197.

Kindig, D. A. (1997). *Purchasing population health: Paying for results*. Ann Arbor, MI: University of Michigan Press.

Kohatsu, N. D., Robinson, J. G., & Torner, J. C. (2004). Evidence-based public health: An evolving concept. *American Journal of Preventive Medicine, 27*(5), 417–421.

National Board of Public Health Examiners. (2010). *National board of public health examiners*. Retrieved on July 20, 2010, from http://www.nbphe.org/about.cfm

Office of the Assistant Secretary for Health and Surgeon General. (1979). *Healthy people: The surgeon general's report on health promotion and disease prevention.* Washington, DC: U.S. Government Printing Office.

Pappas, F., Queen, S., Hadden, W., & Fisher, G. (1993). The increasing disparity in mortality between socioeconomic groups in the United States, 1960 and 1986. *New England Journal of Medicine, 329,* 103–109.

Population Health Institute at the University of Wisconsin. (2010). *County health rankings.* Retrieved July 20, 2010, from http://www.countyhealthrankings.org/health-factors

Public Health Accreditation Board. (2010). *Public health accreditation board.* Retrieved July 10, 2010, from http://www.phaboard.org/

Public Health Foundation. (2010). *Council on linkages: Core competencies for public health professionals.* Retrieved July 20, 2010, from http://www.phf.org/link/corecompetencies.htm#view

Rychetnik, L., Hawe, P., Waters, E., Barratt, A., & Frommer, M. (2004). A glossary for evidence based public health. *Journal of Epidemiology and Community Health, 58,* 538–545.

Sackett, D. L., Straus, S. E., Richardson, W. S., Rosenberg, W., & Haynes, R. B. (2000). *Evidence-based medicine: How to practice and teach EBM.* Churchill Livingstone, New York.

Schwartz, E., Kofie, V. Y., Rivo, M., & Tuckson, R. V. (1990). Black/White comparisons of deaths preventable by medical interventions. *International Journal of Epidemiology, 19,* 591–598.

Tilson, H. H. (2008). Public health accreditation: Progress on national accountability. *Annual Review of Public Health, 29,* xv–xxii.

United Nations International Children's Emergency Fund. (2010). *Definitions: Basic indicators.* Retrieved October 25, 2010, from http://www.unicef.org/infobycountry/stats_popup1.html

U.S. Census Bureau. (2005). *Statistical abstract of the United States: 2006.* Washington, DC: U.S. Department of Commerce.

U.S. Department of Health and Human Services. (2000). *Healthy people 2010: Understanding and improving health* (2nd ed.). Washington, DC: U.S. Government Printing Office.

U.S. Department of Health and Human Services. (2010). *Phase I report recommendations for the framework and format of healthy people 2020.* Retrieved July 20, 2010, from http://www.healthypeople.gov/hp2020/advisory/PhaseI/sec3.htm

World Health Organization. (2006a). *Healthy life expectancy (HALE) at birth (years).* Retrieved October 25, 2010, from http://www.who.int/whosis/indicators/2007HALE0/en/

World Health Organization. (2006b). *Life tables for WHO member states.* Retrieved January 5, 2007, from http://www.who.int/whosis/en/

7

Public Health: Promise and Prospects

Throughout this book, we have referred to public health's mission, articulated by the Institute of Medicine's (IOM) Committee for the Study of the Future of Public Health (IOM, 1988), as the promise of public health:

The broad mission of public health is to "fulfill society's interest in assuring conditions in which people can be healthy" (IOM, 1988, p. 1).

The promise of public health, then, is the assurance that the context in which people live their lives will promote health. Public health, as a field and as a collection of professionals, aspires to provide people with the opportunity to be healthy by ensuring that environments, in the broadest sense, advance health. Healthy communities! Healthy cities! Healthy workplaces! Healthy schools! Each of these phrases, which are often rallying cries for public health, expresses the aspirations of public health to create healthful environments.

Thus, the cornerstone of public health practice is prevention, particularly primary prevention, whereby disease and injury do not occur. Prevention is public health's historic and ideal approach to promoting health, and the distinguishing public health prevention strategy is to influence the "conditions" (i.e., the environment in the fullest sense) in which people live.

"Social justice is the foundation of public health" (Krieger & Birn, 1998, p. 1603), and the commitment to social justice defines the "public health sensibility." Public health assumes that all people are deserving of conditions that promote health—not just the rich, but people of all incomes; not only the young or the old, but also people of all ages; not exclusively the majority race or ethnic group, but people of all races and ethnicities. Public health is a leader and plays an integral role in carrying out this societal

223

obligation to ensure that all people have the opportunity to be healthy. For this reason, public health is often associated with advocating and providing health services for the structurally disadvantaged—those with the least power, wealth, and status—in their social circumstances.

Indeed, public health practice may be thought of as applied social justice.

HAS PUBLIC HEALTH LIVED UP TO ITS IDEAL?

Gross indicators of public health success include increasing life expectancy; decreasing rates of premature death; decreasing rates of disease, injury, and disability among the young; and decreasing rates of preventable health problems such as injuries. We discussed some of these indicators in Chapter 6, finding that public health in the United States has had successes, but serious failures, as well.

An encouraging finding was the drop in age-adjusted premature death rates for many leading causes of death between 1980 and 2006 (National Center for Health Statistics [NCHS], 2010, table 27). Overall, years of potential life lost declined for diseases of the heart including ischemic heart disease, malignant neoplasms, cerebrovascular diseases, influenza and pneumonia, chronic liver disease and cirrhosis, human immunodeficiency virus (HIV), unintentional injuries including motor vehicle–related injuries, suicide, and homicide. Years of potential life lost before age 75 from diseases of the heart declined from 2,238.7 years per 100,000 population in 1980 to 1,077.8 years per 100,000 population in 2006. Years lost to malignant neoplasms decreased from 2,108.8 to 1,490.5, and this included declines in lung, colorectal, prostate, and breast cancer. The only increases in years of potential life lost between 1980 and 2006 came from diabetes mellitus, chronic lower respiratory diseases, and unintentional injuries caused by poisoning. On a percentage basis, loss of potential years of life for males declined more than for women (34% versus 27%). Although the starting point was so much worse for males (13,777 years versus 7,350 years in 1980), males still had more potential years of life lost than females in 2006 (9,092 versus 5,364). Overall declines in years of potential life lost were similar for Whites, Blacks, and Native Americans by around 34%.

Thus, looking at the overall improvement in premature death suggests that efforts have been successful. However, the rate of premature death and years of potential life lost still remained higher for Blacks and Native Americans than for Whites in 2006, at 11,646 years, 8,517 years, and 6,713 years, respectively. These disparities indicate that conditions that produce health remain unequal.

In addition, the United States does poorly on most indicators compared to other highly developed nations including life expectancy, infant mortality, and premature-death. Most importantly, health disparities within the United States indicate that some people have not been provided with the same opportunities to be healthy as others, particularly Blacks, Hispanics, and Native Americans, and the poor. For example, years of potential life lost in 2006 was 985 years per 100,000 population for Whites and 1,969 years per 100,000 population for Blacks. Furthermore, the rates for years of potential life lost per 100,000 population were 158 and 431 years for cerebrovascular diseases for Whites and Blacks, respectively; 1,456 for Whites and 2,003 years for Blacks for malignant neoplasms; and 155 and 375 years for diabetes mellitus for Whites and Blacks, respectively (NCHS, 2010, table 27).

Life expectancy, premature death rates, and so forth are outcome measures of public health performance, but we can also examine process indicators, that is, the practices of public health in the United States. Does public health practice produce the "conditions" that people need to be healthy? If we take physical health[1]—infectious and noninfectious diseases and injury—we might say that there are certain physical requirements and tangible services needed to ensure health. These would include adequate and safe housing; safe workplaces; nutritious and toxin-free food; clean air and water; safe transportation; opportunities for exercise and recreation; and access to quality health care. The public health system, including formal public health—the federal, state, and local health agencies that provide public health leadership and services—the nongovernmental organizations (NGOs), and private partner organizations, address all of these conditions to varying degrees and with varying success.

For example, there is a strong and effective infectious disease prevention effort that includes development of vaccines, vaccination programs, processes for maintaining a food and water supply free from infectious

---

[1] Although mental health and physical health are highly correlated, public health is not as active in mental health prevention and control, and this issue will not be taken up here.

disease agents, and surveillance of emerging diseases. The infectious disease rates reflect the effectiveness, by and large, of this prevention effort. AIDS provides an instructive illustration. AIDS, when first diagnosed in the 1980s, was a "death sentence" for those who contracted it—largely homosexual men, intravenous drug users and their partners, children of infected mothers, and hemophiliacs. A massive effort to understand the disease etiology, develop treatments, and prevent spread was undertaken, and this effort has been quite successful. By the late 1990s, AIDS diagnoses and deaths related to AIDS began to decline sharply primarily because of the success of highly active antiretroviral therapies introduced in 1996 (Centers for Disease Control and Prevention [CDC], 2010a; Osmond, 2003). However, the decline was not uniform across all groups of people with HIV/AIDS.

> The greatest disparity in rates of persons living with AIDS and persons dying of AIDS is that between black men and white men. Although more than a third (34%) of persons living with AIDS in 2000 were white men, this group accounted for only 19% of deaths. In contrast, black men accounted for 42% of persons living with AIDS and 57% of AIDS deaths. (CDC, 2010a, Mortality Trends, para. 6)

These disparities were the result primarily of differences in access to testing and treatment.

WHAT ARE THE BARRIERS TO PUBLIC HEALTH IN MEETING ITS MISSION?

The public health mission to provide people with conditions in which they can be healthy runs counter to the very strong orientation in the United States toward individual accountability and responsibility for one's own actions and situation. Changing the environment to change behavior is less consistent with the value of individual accountability than attempting to hold the individual accountable for his or her own behavior. For example, the view that obesity in the United States should be reduced by changing an environment that encourages weight loss, rather than by educating and motivating people to lose weight themselves, is not an acceptable strategy to many. They view the problem of obesity as one of individual motivation, rather than as a situational determinant. Reducing access to sweetened beverages, providing convenient places to exercise, and structuring grocery store food selections—some of the current public health strategies to reduce the prevalence of obesity (Khan et al., 2009)—are less preferable than strategies that emphasize individual responsibility for food and physical activity choices.

However, public health is increasingly favoring the view that changes to the environment have the most influence on health and must be included in public health prevention strategies. Referring back to the health impact pyramid discussed in Chapter 1, Frieden (2010), Director of the CDC, states that changes in socioeconomic factors such as reduction in poverty and increased education have the greatest impact on health. This bottom layer is followed in impact by "changing the context to make individuals' default decisions healthy" (p. 591).

As another example, obesity is strongly related to onset of noninfectious diseases including cardiovascular disease, stroke, and diabetes. Obesity rates have risen steadily since the 1970s.

> Between 1976–1980 and 2005–2006, the prevalence of overweight among preschool-age children 2–5 years of age more than doubled, from 5% to 11%. . . . Among adults 20–74 years of age, obesity rates have more than doubled since 1976–1980. From 1976–1980 to 2005–2006, the percentage of adults who were obese increased from 15% to 35% (age adjusted). (NCHS, 2010, p. 7)

As we saw in Chapter 5, the CDC-recommended community strategies to prevent obesity (Khan et al., 2009) are heavily weighted to changing the environment by limiting access to sweetened beverages, increasing availability of healthier food and beverage choices in public service venues, improving the geographic availability of supermarkets in underserved areas, and providing incentives to food retailers to locate in and/or offer healthier food and beverage choices in underserved areas.

In addition to clashing with cultural values associated with individualism, the development of the public health system as a predominantly government endeavor goes against a strong conservative segment of the population that prefers the private over the public sector in all societal activities. This explains much of the collaboration between public, private, and nongovernmental nonprofit organizations in public health today. The private sector is strong and rich. Conflict, compromise, and the weakening of public health initiatives have resulted when private interests and the public good are not aligned. Moreover, the 2010 Supreme Court ruling that lifts limits on corporate spending for elections (Citizens United v Federal Election Commission, 130 S.Ct. 876 (2010)) will make the private sector even more powerful.

The 2009 health care reform legislation is an example of the power of the private sector to influence public health policy for its own well-being, in this case, for insurance companies. The legislation does not have a public option, as public health would have preferred. It maintains and promotes the mixed pubic/private system of health care coverage with continued and expanded participation by health insurance companies, adding inefficiencies, difficulty with oversight, administrative costs, and complexities of the new system. As a result, the health care reform bill is not optimal, and even President Obama admits that it will need revision in the coming years. However, the legislation was the compromise reached to get a bill of any kind because of the influence of the private sector.

The history of efforts to prevent lead exposure provides another example of the difficulty of achieving public health goals when private sector interests are threatened.

> The history of child lead poisoning in the past century is a good example of how powerful economic interest can prevent the implementation of a useful truth. . . . In 1786 Benjamin Franklin listed in a letter to a friend every profession for which lead posed a health hazard. He then predicted that years would pass before the truth of a public health tragedy would be confronted. In fact, long after the lead and lead paint industries became aware of the hazards posed by lead, particularly in young children, they continued to market their products aggressively. They lobbied legislatures to stall all regulation, suppressed research findings, and advertised falsely and in doing so created a problem that grew to major proportions over decades. Benjamin Franklin's prediction proved correct. (DeBuono, 2006, p. 41)

Public health efforts to reduce exposure to lead continued with battles to remove lead from paint, manufacturing processes, and especially gasoline, to which it had been added since the mid-1940s:

> In 1986, a complete ban finally took effect and all gasoline was unleaded. This was successful in reducing child blood lead level. Before the ban was implemented, 88% of children in the United States had blood levels higher than 10 ug/dl. Afterwards, only 9% had elevated blood levels. The blood lead levels of all Americans declined 78% between 1978 and 1991,

falling in exact proportion to the declining levels of lead in the overall gas online supply. As a result of EPA's regulatory efforts to remove lead from gasoline between 1980 and 1999 emission of lead from the transportation sector declined by 95% and levels of lead in the air decreased by 94%. Following years of heated debate, congress banned lead based paints for use in housing in 1978. By the time, the ban went into effect, the industry no longer opposed the ban, reeling from negative publicity and a precipitous decline in sales of lead based paint. (DeBuono, 2006, p. 44)

The story of public health's difficulty in controlling exposure to lead is not unique. Efforts to prevent exposure to other disease-producing substances including cigarettes, pesticides such as dichlorodiphenyltrichloroethane (DDT), mercury in vaccines and manufacturing processes, and carbon monoxide are much the same. Removal of DDT from the environment is another instructive story. Rachel Carson, who wrote *Silent Spring* in 1962, was a trained marine biologist, and her book became a "call to arms" for the environmental movement. Unlike other insecticides that were narrow in their targets, DDT killed hundreds of species at once. Carson observed the effects of DDT on wildlife, particularly how damaging it was to the eggshells of raptors such as eagles, falcons, and hawks, leading to a significant decline in their population, which, in turn, reverberated through the ecosystem. Although *Silent Spring*'s message was powerful enough to lead to a public demand for a ban on DDT, the government began with an increase in oversight on DDT use. It was not until 1972 that the Environmental Protection Agency (EPA) instituted a total ban, a major victory for the environmental movement.

The chemical industry, led by Monsanto, characterized Carson's findings as one sided for failing to point out how pesticides had eliminated malaria, typhus, and other human scourges. (These industrial attacks were and are common in the tobacco, oil, and chemical industries.) The chemical industry suffered a backlash when the public recognized Carson's solid research and their interconnectedness of the natural environment (Cox, 2000).

Carson earned a reputation as a careful researcher and compelling author. In the 1950s, she wrote two popular books, *The Sea Around Us* and *The Edge of the Sea*, introducing the general public to ecology.

The history of community health centers is another example of major reform in public health that succeeded in spite of strong opposition (Lefkowitz, 2007). Community health centers were developed by H. Jack Geiger in the 1970s with grassroots support, beginning from one center in Mississippi and growing eventually to more than a thousand. They were intended to serve those without resources or advantages—the poor and powerless. They addressed health and social problems comprehensively including health care services, housing, food, job creation, and education. They offered comprehensive services for health improvement. Geiger saw them as necessary for social justice. Public financing of the community health centers was opposed by conservative legislators who held to individual accountability. Community health centers were originally implemented as a pilot project with slight funding. With their success, they gained federal funding, although, in the more conservative Reagan era, their budgets were constrained and the scope of their activities became limited to health care.

GLOBAL HEALTH THREATS AND PUBLIC HEALTH IN THE UNITED STATES

As we look about the world today, there are many potential threats to global health that will affect or have affected health in the United States, directly or indirectly. These include infectious disease pandemics, worldwide water and food shortages, climate change, declining air quality, and environmental degradation from population growth and industrialization.

Not surprisingly, public health in the United States and worldwide has the leadership role in infectious disease prevention and control. Trends in movement throughout the globe have brought increased and more rapid transmission of infectious disease agents. More people are traveling internationally more frequently than ever before. An example of the consequences of current travel patterns is the rapid spread of SARS (severe acute respiratory syndrome), an infectious disease transmitted by person-to-person contact, which began in Asia in February 2003 and spread within several months to more than two dozen countries in North America, South America, Europe, and Asia before it was controlled. A total of 8,098 persons contracted SARS during 2003, and 774 died (CDC, 2010c). Global infectious disease outbreaks are a serious threat, and public health, principally through the World Health Organization (WHO), the CDC, and their partner organizations throughout the world provide leadership in the prevention and control of infectious disease spread through continual monitoring and development of responses.

With regard to other emerging and serious threats to health such as climate change, water and food shortages, and environmental degradation, public health's role has been to advocate for primary prevention, but to put most efforts into providing or preparing for secondary and tertiary prevention. That is, the public health system in the United States is involved more in responding to the consequences of these threats than in trying to prevent them. For example, the CDC describes its response to climate change as follows:

> To lead efforts to anticipate, prevent and respond to the broad range of effects on the health of Americans and the nation's public health infrastructure. CDC's expertise and programs in environmental health, infectious disease, and other fields form the foundation of public health efforts in preparedness for climate change. (CDC, 2010b, para. 1)

Another present and serious threat to health worldwide is war. The health consequences of war are staggering, not just in terms of the injury, disability, and death of combatants, but in terms of civilian morbidity, mortality, and displacement. Destruction of civil societies through war and the flood of refugees that often ensues are a public health problem of major proportions.

There are also what are called Black Swan events such as massive industrial accidents that have direct and indirect health consequences. Black Swan events (Taleb, 2007) are described as extremely high impact with low probability of occurrence. The 2010 British Petroleum (BP) oil leak from a deepwater well in the Gulf of Mexico and the 1986 Chernobyl nuclear accident are examples of Black Swans. These and natural disasters such as Hurricane Katrina are threats to health that have huge impacts on public health and should be incorporated into public health practice.

Public health in the United States must participate optimally with partners throughout the world to the global efforts to prevent and control the adverse consequences of these threats.

CHALLENGES FOR PUBLIC HEALTH

In the United States, there are compelling cultural values and preferences for individualism and the private sector, which support powerful interests that favor the status quo and constrain the ability to change the environment in ways that would promote health. Thus, these values and preferences work against an optimally effective public health system. Therefore, having the skills to bring about change within this context are essential for public health professionals if we are to realize public health's potential to control and prevent disease, injury, and premature death in the United States. Grassroots support and mobilization are vital. Public health professionals must develop organizing capabilities to mobilize communities, regions, and populations to fight for the conditions they need to ensure health for all. These conditions that produce health include, at a minimum, adequate and safe housing; safe workplaces; nutritious and toxin-free food; clean air and drinking water; safe transportation; opportunities for exercise and recreation; and access to quality health care. They must also include sustaining incomes for all and education that prepares all adults for meaningful participation in the economy. Finally, public health in the United States must participate in the reduction and prevention of global health problems, both because these affect health in the United States and because doing so is consistent with the "public health sensibility."

REFERENCES

Centers for Disease Control and Prevention. (2010a). *AIDS trends and HIV/AIDS mortality*. Retrieved August 10, 2010, from http://www.cdc.gov/hiv/topics/surveillance/resources/guidelines/epi-guideline/la_supp/section1q2_trends.htm

Centers for Disease Control and Prevention. (2010b). *Climate change and public health*. Retrieved August 10, 2010, from http://www.cdc.gov/climatechange/

Centers for Disease Control and Prevention. (2010c). *Severe acute respiratory syndrome (SARS)*. Retrieved August 20, 2010, from http://www.cdc.gov/ncidod/sars/factsheet.htm

Citizens United v Federal Election Commission, 130 S.Ct. 876 (2010)

Cox, S. (2000). *The industrial evolution: Creating a foundation of corporate sustainability*. Retrieved October 27, 2010, from www.me.sc.edu/Research/lss/Papers/ShannonThesis.pdf

DeBuono, B. A. (editor). (2006). *Milestones in Public Health*. New York: Pfizer Global Pharmaceuticals.

Frieden, T. R. (2010). A framework for public health action: The health impact pyramid. *American Journal of Public Health, 100*(4), 590–595.

Institute of Medicine. (1988). *The future of public health*. Washington, DC: National Academy Press.

Khan, L. K., Sobush, K., Keener, D., Goodman, K., Lowry, A., Kakietek, J., et al. (2009). Recommended community strategies and measurements to prevent obesity in the United States. *Morbidity and Mortality Weekly Report, 58*, 1–26.

Krieger, N., & Birn, A. E. (1998). A vision of social justice as the foundation of public health: Commemorating 150 years of the spirit of 1848. *American Journal of Public Health, 88*(11), 1603–1606.

Lefkowitz, B. (2007). *Community Health Centers: A Movement and the People Who Made It Happen.* New Brunswick, NJ: Rutgers University Press.

National Center for Health Statistics. (2010). *Health, United States, 2009.* Hyattsville, MD: Department of Health and Human Services.

Osmond, D.H. (2003). Epidemiology of HIV/AIDS in the United States. *HIV InSite.* Retrieved August 10, 2010, from http://hivinsite.ucsf.edu/InSite?page=kb-01-03

Taleb, N. N. (2007). *The Black Swan: The Impact of the Highly Improbable.* New York: Random House.

Index

Note: Page numbers followed by *f* indicate figures and *t* indicate tables.